PATIENT ASSESSMENT HANDBOOK

RICHARD A. CHERRY, M.S., NREMT-P
Assistant Emergency Medicine Residency Director

Prentice Hall

UPPER SADDLE RIVER, NEW JERSEY 07458

Library of Congress Cataloging-in-Publication Data
Cherry, Richard A.
    Patient assessment handbook / Richard A. Cherry
        p. cm.
    Includes bibliographical references and index.
    ISBN 0-13-061578-1
    1. Diagnosis—Handbooks, manuals, etc.   2. Medical history taking—Handbooks,
manuals, etc.   3. Physical diagnosis—Handbooks, manuals, etc.   4. Neurologic
examination—Handbooks, manuals, etc.   I. Title.

RC71 .C556   2002
616.07'5-dc21   2001036555

Publisher: Julie Levin Alexander
Acquisition Editor: Greg Vis
Managing Development Editor: Lois Berlowitz
Director of Production and Manufacturing: Bruce Johnson
Managing Production Editor: Patrick Walsh
Marketing Manager: Tiffany Price
Editorial / production supervision and interior design: Inkwell Publishing Services
Design Director: Cheryl Asherman
Design Coordinator: Maria Guglielmo-Walsh
Cover Photography: Eddie Sperling Photography
Cover Illustration: Malcolm Farley
Manufacturing Buyer: Pat Brown
Printer / Binder: Banta Viking

10 9 8 7 6 5 4 3 2 1
ISBN 0-13-061578-1

NOTICE ON CARE PROCEDURES

It is the intent of the authors and publisher that this handbook be used as part of a formal EMT-Paramedic program taught by qualified instructors and supervised by a licensed physician. The procedures described in this handbook are based upon consultation with EMT and medical authorities. The authors and publisher have taken care to make certain that these procedures reflect currently accepted clinical practice; however, they cannot be considered absolute recommendations.

The material in this handbook contains the most current information available at the time of publication. However, federal, state, and local guidelines concerning clinical practices, including, without limitation, those governing infection control and universal precautions, change rapidly. The reader should note, therefore, that the new regulations may require changes in some procedures.

It is the responsibility of the reader to familiarize himself or herself with the policies and procedures set by federal, state, and local agencies as well as the institution or agency where the reader is employed. The authors and publisher of this handbook disclaim any liability, loss, or risk resulting directly or indirectly from the suggested procedures and theory, from any undetected errors, or from the reader's misunderstanding of the text. It is the reader's responsibility to stay informed of any new changes or recommendations made by any federal, state, and local agency as well as by his or her employing institution or agency.

CONTENTS

TAKING A HISTORY

THE PHYSICAL EXAM

THE NEUROLOGICAL EXAM

EMERGENCY FIELD ASSESSMENTS

APPENDICES

REVIEWERS

The following instructors provided many excellent suggestions in the development of this handbook. The quality of their reviews is outstanding, and their assistance is greatly appreciated.

Stephen J. Rahm, NREMT-P
EMT Program Coordinator
Ft. Sam Houston, Texas

Douglas Stevenson, B.A., NREMT-P
Alvin Community College
Alvin, Texas

Eric Stokely, A.A.S., EMT-P
Emergency Medical Technology
Holmes Community College
Snellville, Georgia

TAKING A HISTORY

ESTABLISHING RAPPORT

MAKE A GOOD FIRST IMPRESSION

When you arrive on the scene, your patient, his family, and bystanders will form an impression of you. You only have a few precious minutes to make that impression a positive one. Present yourself as a caring, compassionate, competent, and confident health care professional. Your voice, body language, gestures, and especially eye contact should communicate that you care about your patient's problems. A calm, reassuring voice and demeanor can put even the most apprehensive patient at ease.

INTRODUCE YOURSELF

As you enter, make immediate eye contact with your patient and maintain it as you conduct the interview. Introduce yourself by name, title, and agency. Be aware of other nonverbal forms of communication. Your tone of voice, facial expressions, and body language convey your true attitudes. Touch is a powerful communication tool. Used properly, it conveys compassion, caring, and reassurance to your already apprehensive patient.

ASK THE APPROPRIATE QUESTIONS

To gather the patient history, use a combination of open-ended and closed-ended questions. Open-ended questions such as "Can you describe the pain in your chest?" allow your patient to respond freely and without limits. Closed-ended questions elicit a short answer to a very direct question. They are appropriate when time or your patient's mental status or condition doesn't allow for open-ended questions. For example, if your patient is gasping for breath while you're trying to determine the cause, phrase your questions for one-word answers or yes-no nods.

USE APPROPRIATE LANGUAGE

Nothing distances you from your patient more quickly than using sophisticated medical terminology. Most of your patients will not understand medical terms. For effective communication to occur, you and your patient must understand each other.

ACTIVE LISTENING TECHNIQUES

FACILITATION
Maintain sincere eye contact, use concerned facial gestures, and lean forward while you listen. Saying "Mm-hmm" or "Go on" or "I'm listening" help your patient open up.

REFLECTION
Repeat your patient's words. This encourages him to provide more details. Just make sure not to disturb his train of thought.

CLARIFICATION
Patients often cannot clearly describe what they feel. They often will use vague and general words. Do not hesitate to ask for clarification.

EMPATHY
Show empathy by responding with "I understand" or "That must have been very difficult." Sometimes just a gesture like handing him a tissue or patting him on the shoulder conveys empathy.

CONFRONTATION
If you detect inconsistencies in your patient's story, confront him with your observations. For example: "You say your chest doesn't hurt but you keep rubbing it." Confrontation may help your patient bring his hidden feelings into the open.

INTERPRETATION
Question your patient about what you believe may be the problem. For example: "You say your chest doesn't hurt, but you keep rubbing it. Are you afraid you are having a heart attack but don't want to admit it?" This technique further demonstrates empathy.

ASKING ABOUT FEELINGS
Ask your patient how he feels about what he is experiencing. Showing genuine interest in his problem may unlock the door to key information that he otherwise may not have shared with you.

THE COMPREHENSIVE HISTORY

Components of a Comprehensive History

- Preliminary Data
- Chief Complaint
- Present Illness
- Past History
- Current Health Status
- Review of Systems

PRELIMINARY DATA

Determine your patient's age, sex, race, birthplace, and occupation. Evaluate the reliability of the source of the information. Is it the competent patient himself, his spouse, a friend, a bystander, a first responder, the police, or another health care worker? Do you have the medical record from a transferring facility? Are you taking report from a reliable first responder?

CHIEF COMPLAINT

The chief complaint is the pain, discomfort, or dysfunction that caused your patient to request help. Begin with a general question that allows your patient to respond freely. For example: "Why did you call us today?" or "What seems to be the problem?" When possible, report and record the chief complaint in your patient's own words. For example: "I am having a hard time breathing" or "My chest hurts." For the unconscious patient, the chief complaint becomes what someone else said, or what you observed as the primary problem. For example, in some trauma situations, the chief complaint might be the mechanism of injury such as "a gunshot wound to the chest" or "a fall from 25 feet."

PRESENT ILLNESS

Once you have determined the chief complaint, explore each of your patient's complaints in greater detail. A practical template for exploring each complaint follows the mnemonic OPQRST–ASPN.

ONSET

Did the problem develop suddenly or gradually? What was your patient doing when the symptoms started? In medical emergencies, investigate your patient's activities at the time of, or shortly before, the signs or symptoms developed. Was the patient exercising or exerting himself, or at rest or sleeping? Was he eating or drinking? If so, what? In trauma cases, assure that a medical problem did not cause the accident. For example, the sudden onset of an illness such as a seizure or syncope may have caused a fall.

PROVOCATION

What provokes the symptom or alleviates it? Ask your patient how position or breathing affects the discomfort. If your patient took a medication shortly before you arrived, its effect or lack of effect may help determine the problem. Investigate any medication used to relieve a problem, and note its effectiveness. Ask about any activity, medication, or other circumstance that either alleviates or aggravates the chief complaint.

QUALITY

Investigate how your patient perceives the pain or discomfort. Ask him to explain how the symptom feels, and listen carefully to his answer. Does your patient call his pain crushing, tearing, oppressive, gnawing, crampy, sharp, dull, or otherwise? Quote his descriptors in your report.

REGION/RADIATION

Identify the exact location and area of pain, discomfort, or dysfunction. Does your patient complain of pain "here," while holding a clenched fist over the sternum, or does he grasp the entire abdomen with both hands and moan? Ask your patient to point to the painful area. Identify the specific location, or the boundary of the pain if it is regional. Determine whether the pain moves or radiates. Evaluate moving pain as to its initial location, progression, and any factors that affect its movement. Note any pain that may be referred from another part of the body.

SEVERITY

How bad is the symptom? Ask him how bad the pain feels, and then have him compare it to other painful problems he has experienced. Ask him to describe the severity of the pain on a scale from 1 to 10, 10 being the worst pain he has ever felt. Also notice the amount of discomfort your patient's condition causes. Is your patient very still and resistive to your touch? Is he writhing about?

TIME

When did the symptoms begin? Is it constant or intermittent? How long does it last? How long has this symptom affected your patient? When did any previous episodes occur? Does this episode vary in length from earlier ones?

ASSOCIATED SYMPTOMS

What other symptoms commonly associated with the chief complaint in certain diseases can help rule in your field diagnosis? For example, if the chief complaint is chest pain, ask "Are you short of breath? Are you nauseous? Have you vomited? Are you dizzy or light-headed?"

PERTINENT NEGATIVES

A pertinent negative is the absence of a finding that might be expected to be associated with your patient's problem. The absence of associated symptoms is as important to the diagnosis as the presence of them because the absence helps rule out certain diagnoses. Note any element of the history or physical exam that does not support a suspected or possible diagnosis.

PAST HISTORY

The past history may provide you with significant insight into your patient's chief complaint and your diagnosis. Look in depth at the following:

GENERAL STATE OF HEALTH

How does your patient perceive his general state of health?

CHILDHOOD DISEASES

What childhood diseases did he have? Did he have mumps, measles, rubella, whooping cough, chicken pox, rheumatic fever, scarlet fever, or polio?

ADULT DISEASES

Has your patient recently seen a physician or been hospitalized? If so, for what conditions? If you discover a pre-existing medical problem, investigate its effects on your patient. When was he last affected by the problem? Is your patient on any special diets, taking prescribed medications, or restricted in activity?

PSYCHIATRIC ILLNESSES

Does your patient have a history of mental illness? Has he ever been diagnosed with depression, mania, schizophrenia, etc.? Is he being treated for a mental illness? If so, what medications is he taking? Has he ever had thoughts of suicide? Has he ever attempted suicide?

ACCIDENTS OR INJURIES

Has your patient ever had a serious accident or injury requiring hospitalization? Has he had a previous injury that could be a factor in his current problem? Keep this line of questioning to relevant information only.

SURGERIES OR HOSPITALIZATIONS

Ask your patient if there were any other hospitalizations or surgeries not already mentioned.

CURRENT HEALTH STATUS

The current health status assembles all the factors in your patient's medical condition. Try to gather information that completes the puzzle surrounding your patient's primary problem.

CURRENT MEDICATIONS

Is your patient taking any medications? This includes over-the-counter, prescribed, home remedies, vitamins, and minerals. If so, why? A recently prescribed medication may cause an allergic or untoward reaction. It also may be out of date and no longer effective.

ALLERGIES

Ask your patient about any known allergies, especially those to penicillin, the "caine" family (local anesthetics), or tetanus toxoid. These agents are occasionally given in emergency situations. Find out what type of reaction your patient had to it. For example, was it just a mild allergic reaction with a rash and some itching, or some localized swelling, or anaphylactic shock? Knowledge of your patient's allergies may prevent additional complications during the emergency department visit, especially if he becomes disoriented or unconscious during transport. If your patient is short of breath with wheezing, ask about environmental allergies. In cases of possible anaphylaxis, ask about allergies to foods (e.g., shellfish, nuts, and dairy products) and insect bites and stings.

TOBACCO

Does your patient use tobacco? If so, what (cigarettes, cigars, pipe, smokeless, etc.), how much, and for how long? To quantify his smoking history, multiply the number of packs per day smoked by the number of years. The result is his pack/year history. For example, if your patient smoked 2 packs of cigarettes per day for 25 years, he is a 50 pack/year smoker. A number over 30 pack/years is considered significant.

ALCOHOL, DRUGS, AND RELATED SUBSTANCES

Alcohol and drugs are often contributing factors, if not the cause, of your patient's medical problems. Gather data that will help direct your patient's medical treatment. Remaining nonjudgmental will aid you in your questioning. Start with a general question such as "How much alcohol do you drink?" If you suspect a drinking problem may be a factor, use the **CAGE** questionnaire (an alcoholism screening instrument) to determine the presence of alcoholism.

The CAGE Questionnaire

C   Have you ever felt the need to **Cut** down on your drinking?

A   Have you ever felt **Annoyed** by criticism of your drinking?

G   Have you ever had **Guilty** feelings about drinking?

E   Have you ever taken a drink first thing in the morning as an **Eye-opener**?

Two or more "Yes" answers suggest alcoholism and further lines of inquiry. Ask about blackouts, accidents, or injuries that happened while drinking. Also ask about alcohol-related job losses, marital problems, and arrests while under the influence of alcohol. Similarly, ask about drug use. For example: "Do you use marijuana, cocaine, heroin, sleeping pills, painkillers?" "How much do you take?" "How do these drugs make you feel?" "Have you had any bad reactions?"

DIET

Ask about your patient's normal daily intake of food and drink. Are there any dietary restrictions or supplements? Also ask about the use of foods with stimulating effects such as coffee, tea, cola drinks, and other beverages containing caffeine.

SCREENING TESTS

Inquire about PPD (Pure Protein Derivative) tests for suspected tuberculosis; Pap smears and mammograms; stool testing for occult blood; and cholesterol tests. Record the dates of the tests and their results.

IMMUNIZATIONS

Ask your patient about his immunizations for diseases such as tetanus, pertussis, diphtheria, polio, measles, rubella, mumps, influenza, hepatitis B, *Hemophilus influenza* type B, and pneumococcal vaccine.

SLEEP PATTERNS

Ask your patient what time he normally goes to bed and arises. Does he take daytime naps? Does he have problems falling asleep or staying asleep?

EXERCISE AND LEISURE ACTIVITIES

Does your patient exercise regularly or lead a sedentary lifestyle? Sometimes your patient's lifestyle will support your diagnosis.

ENVIRONMENTAL HAZARDS

Ask about possible hazards in the home, in school, and at the workplace. For example, your patient may live in an area with high levels of toxic substances. Many health problems can be traced to these environmental causes.

USE OF SAFETY MEASURES

In an auto accident, did your patient use a seat restraint system? Were all passengers belted in? Did the air bag deploy? This type of information aids you and the emergency department staff in determining the extent of damage caused by a particular mechanism of injury. For bicycle, roller blade, and skateboard injuries, ask about the use of helmets, knee and elbow pads.

FAMILY HISTORY

In the nonemergency setting you may explore deep into the family tree and chart the medical history of grandparents, parents, aunts, and uncles. In the emergency setting, learning that your 45-year-old chest pain patient's father and brother both died of heart attacks in their late forties is important information. Look for incidence of diabetes, heart disease, hypercholesterolemia, high blood pressure, stroke, kidney disease, tuberculosis, cancer, arthritis, anemia, allergies, asthma, headaches, epilepsy, mental illness, alcoholism, drug addiction, and any symptoms like your patient's.

HOME SITUATION AND SIGNIFICANT OTHERS

Ask your patient who lives at home with him. Ask him about his home life, or lack of one. Ask about friends, family, support groups, loved ones. Find out if he has a support network and whom it includes. Who takes care of him when he needs help? Loneliness and isolation may complicate your patient's physical symptoms.

DAILY LIFE

Ask your patient to describe his typical day. When does he get up? What does he do first? Then what? These types of questions reveal a lot about your patient's state of mind and general wellness. Is he busy, active, and motivated to get up in the morning? Does he merely exist from the time he awakens and go through life with no purpose or direction? Is he under high levels of stress from morning to night in a job that requires him to take his problems home with him?

IMPORTANT EXPERIENCES

Ask about your patient's upbringing and home life growing up. How much schooling does he have? Was he in the military? What kind of jobs has he held? What is his financial situation? Is he married? Single? Divorced? Widowed? What does he do for fun and relaxation? Is he retired or looking forward to retirement?

RELIGIOUS BELIEFS

Some religions forbid certain treatments and have guidelines regarding the management of illness and injury. For example, some religions forbid administering whole blood to a person.

THE PATIENT'S OUTLOOK

Find out what your patient thinks and how he feels about the present and future.

REVIEW OF SYSTEMS

The review of systems is a series of questions designed to identify problems not already mentioned by your patient. It is a system-by-system list of questions that are more specific than the ones asked during the basic history. The patient's chief complaint, condition, and status determine how much, if any, of the review of systems you will use. Let your patient lead you through the history.

GENERAL

What is your patient's usual weight and have there been any recent weight changes? Has he had weakness, fatigue, or fever?

SKIN

Has he noticed any new rashes, lumps, sores, itching, dryness, color change, or changes in nails or hair? Could cosmetics or jewelry have caused these problems?

HEAD, EYES, EARS, NOSE, AND THROAT (HEENT)

Has he had headaches or recent head trauma? How is his vision? Does he wear glasses or contact lenses? When was his last eye exam? Has he experienced any of the following: pain, redness, excessive tearing, double vision, blurred vision, spots, specks, flashing lights? Has he ever had glaucoma or cataracts? How is his hearing? Does he use hearing aids? Has he ever experienced ringing in the ears (tinnitus), vertigo, earaches, infection, or discharge? Does he get frequent colds, nasal stuffiness, nasal discharge, hay fever, nosebleeds, sinus problems? Does he wear dentures? When was his last dental exam? Describe the condition of his teeth and gums. Do his gums bleed? Does he get a sore tongue, dry mouth, frequent sore throats, or hoarseness? Does he have swollen glands? Has he ever had a goiter, neck pain, or stiffness?

RESPIRATORY

Has he ever had any of the following: wheezing, coughing up blood (hemoptysis), asthma, bronchitis, emphysema, pneumonia, TB, or pleurisy? When was his last chest X-ray? Is he coughing now? If so, can you describe the sputum?

CARDIAC

Has he ever had heart trouble, high blood pressure, rheumatic fever, heart murmurs, chest pain or discomfort, palpitations, shortness of breath, shortness of breath while lying flat, ankle swelling or edema? Has he ever been awakened from sleep with shortness of breath? Has he ever had an ECG or other heart tests?

GASTROINTESTINAL

Has he ever had any of the following: trouble swallowing, heartburn, loss of appetite, nausea/vomiting, regurgitation, vomiting blood, indigestion? How often does he move his bowels? Describe the color and size of his stools. Has there been any changes in his bowel habits? Has he had rectal bleeding or black tarry stools, hemorrhoids, constipation, diarrhea? Has he had abdominal pain, food intolerance, excessive belching or passing of gas? Has he had jaundice, liver or gallbladder problems, or hepatitis?

URINARY

How often does he urinate? Has he ever had any of the following: excessive urination, excessive urination at night, burning or pain while urinating, blood in the urine, urgency, reduced caliber or force of urine flow, hesitancy, dribbling, incontinence? Has he ever had a urinary tract infection or stones?

MALE GENITAL

Has he ever had a hernia, discharge from or sores on the penis, testicular pain, or masses? Has he ever had a sexually transmitted disease? If so, how was it treated?

FEMALE GENITAL

At what age was her first menstrual period? Describe the regularity, frequency, duration, and amount of bleeding of her periods. When was her last menstrual period? Does she bleed between periods or after intercourse? Has she ever had difficulty with her period or premenstrual tension? At what age did she become menopausal? Were there symptoms or bleeding? Has she ever had any of the following: vaginal discharge, lumps, sores, or itching? Has she ever had a sexually transmitted disease? If so, how was it treated? How many times has she been pregnant? How many live deliveries? Any abortions (spontaneous or induced)? Has she ever had complications of pregnancy? Does she use birth control? If so, what type?

PERIPHERAL VASCULAR
Has he ever had intermittent calf pain while walking, leg cramps, varicose veins, or past blood clots?

MUSCULOSKELETAL
Has he ever experienced muscle or joint pain, stiffness, arthritis, gout, or backache? Describe the location or symptoms.

NEUROLOGIC
Has he ever experienced any of the following: fainting, blackouts, seizures, weakness, paralysis, numbness or loss of sensation, tingling, "pins and needles," tremors or other involuntary movements?

HEMATOLOGIC
Has he ever been anemic? Has he ever had a blood transfusion? If so, did he have a reaction to it? Does he bruise or bleed easily?

ENDOCRINE
Has he ever had thyroid trouble? Did he experience heat or cold intolerance, or excessive sweating? Does he have diabetes? Has he ever had excessive thirst, hunger, or urge to urinate?

PSYCHIATRIC
Is he nervous? Is he under much stress and tension? Has he ever been depressed? Has he ever thought of committing suicide?

THE PHYSICAL EXAM

Level of Consciousness
AVPU Scale.

Signs of Distress
Degree of distress, evidence of obvious medical or traumatic problem, pain, or anxiety.

Apparent State of Health
Healthy, robust, vigorous/frail, ill-looking, feeble.

Vital Statistics
Height and weight estimations, general stature, obvious deformities or disproportionate areas, thin or obese.

Sexual Development
Sexual maturity appropriate for age and gender.

Skin Condition
Skin color, lesions, rashes, bruises, scars.

Posture, Gait, Motor Activity
Posture, presentation, positioning, restlessness, involuntary movements.

Personal Grooming
Appropriate dress, shoe alterations, unusual jewelry or medication information tag, appropriate grooming and hygiene.

Odors of Breath or Body
Unusual or striking body or breath odors.

Facial Expression
Facial expressions appropriate for interaction.

Vital Signs
Pulse, BP, respiration, temperature.

PULSE

Exam
Locate and palpate the pulse for rate, quality, and regularity.

Normal
Rate within normal limits for age, strong, and regular.

Age	Range
Newborn	100–180
Infant (<1 yr)	100–160
Toddler (1–2 yrs)	80–110
Preschooler (3–5 yrs)	70–110
School age (6–12 yrs)	65–110
Adolescent (13–18 yrs)	60–90
Adult	60–100

Abnormal

Finding	Significance
Bradycardia	Parasympathetic tone, head injury, hypothermia, severe hypoxia, drug overdose
Tachycardia	Sympathetic tone, blood loss, fear, pain, fever, hypoxia, shock, dysrhythmia
Irregular	Dysrhythmia
Weak	Decreased stroke volume, decreased fluid volume, shock
Bounding	Hypertension, heat stroke, increasing ICP

THE PHYSICAL EXAM

RESPIRATION

Exam

Evaluate breathing for rate, pattern, and quality.

Normal

Rate within normal limits for age, regular pattern, equal depth bilaterally.

Age	Range
Newborn	30–60
Infant (<1 yr)	30–60
Toddler (1–2 yrs)	24–40
Preschooler (3–5 yrs)	22–34
School age (6–12 yrs)	18–30
Adolescent (13–18 yrs)	12–26
Adult	12–20

Abnormal

	Condition	Description
∿∿∿∿∿	Eupnea	Normal breathing rate and pattern
∿∿∿∿∿∿	Tachypnea	Increased respiratory rate
∼∼∼∼	Bradypnea	Decreased respiratory rate
———————	Apnea	Absence of breathing
⋁⋁⋁⋁	Hyperpnea	Normal rate, but deep respirations
᭄ᨏᨏᨏ	Cheyne-Stokes	Gradual increases and decreases in respirations with periods of apnea
ᨏ᭄ᨏ᭄ᨏ	Biot's	Rapid, deep respirations (gasps) with short pauses between sets
ᨏᨏᨏᨏᨏ	Kussmaul's	Tachypnea and hyperpnea
⫽⫽⫽⫽⫽⫽	Apneustic	Prolonged inspiratory phase with shortened expiratory phase

BLOOD PRESSURE

Exam

Evaluate the blood pressure by auscultation, palpation, or doppler.

Normal

BP within normal limits for age.

Age	Range
Newborn	60–90
Infant (<1 yr)	87–105
Toddler (1–2 yrs)	95–105
Preschooler (3–5 yrs)	95–110
School age (6–12 yrs)	97–112
Adolescent (13–18 yrs)	112–128
Adult	Male: 120–150
	Female: 110-150

Abnormal

Finding	Significance
Hypotension	Shock (late)
Hypertension	Head injury, cardiovascular disease, stroke, renal disease
Narrowing pulse pressure	Cardiac tamponade, tension pneumothorax, shock
Widening pulse pressure	Increasing ICP, fever
Orthostatic hypotension	Hypovolemia

BODY TEMPERATURE

Exam
Measure core temperature with a glass thermometer, electronic device, or tympanic membrane device.

Normal
Core temperature under 98.6°F or 37°C.

Abnormal

Finding	Significance
<93°F/34°C	Body systems begin to fail
<90°F/31°C	Thermogenesis stops, cardiac irritability
<70°F/22°C	Irreversible asystole
102°F/38°C	Increase in metabolism
103°F/39°C	Brain neurons denature
>105°F/41°C	Brain cells die, seizures may occur

THE SKIN

Exam
Inspect and palpate the skin for color, temperature, moisture, excessive roughness or thickness, mobility, turgor, and lesions.

Normal
Pink, dry, warm, smooth, good return to normal when pinched, good mobility and turgor, and no lesions.

Abnormal

Finding	Significance
Pale	Hypothermia, shock, anemia
Blue	Hypoxia
Ecchymosis	Bleeding under skin
Jaundice	Liver disease
Excessive dryness	Hypothyroidism, winter side effect
Excessive oiliness	Acne, hyperthyroidism
Sweating	Sympathetic response to anxiety, fear, or exertion
Generalized warming	Environmental, fever, hyperthyroidism
Generalized cooling	Environmental, hypothyroidism
Localized warmth	Bleeding or swelling under skin
Rough	Hypothyroidism
Thin, fragile	Debilitating disease in elderly
Thick	Eczema, psoriasis
Poor turgor	Dehydration
Decreased mobility	Edema, scleroderma

SKIN LESIONS

Exam

Examine the skin for lesions. Describe the following:

A Asymmetry (exact location on the skin's surface)

B Border—size in centimeters, shape (oval, spherical, irregular, tubular), mobility (movable, fixed)

C Color, configuration, consistency (hard, soft, edematous, cystic, nodular)

D Diameter (length, width, depth) and drainage

Vascular Lesions

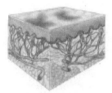

Purpura—Reddish-purple blotches, diameter more than 0.5 cm

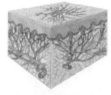

Spider angioma—Reddish legs radiate from red spot

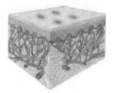

Petechiae—Reddish-purple spots, diameter less than 0.5 cm

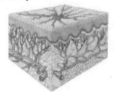

Venous star—Bluish legs radiate from blue center

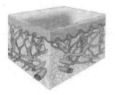

Ecchymoses—Reddish-purple blotch, size varies

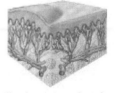

Capillary hemangioma—Irregular red spots

Primary Lesions

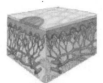

Macule—Flat spot, color varies from white to brown or from red to purple, diameter less than 1 cm

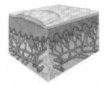

Plaque—Superficial papule, diameter more than 1 cm, rough texture

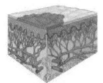

Patch—Irregular flat macule, diameter greater than 1 cm

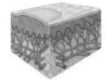

Wheal—Pink, irregular spot varying in size and shape

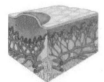

Papule—Elevated firm spot, color varies from brown to red or from pink to purplish red, diameter less than 1 cm

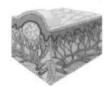

Nodule—Elevated firm spot, diameter 1–2 cm

Primary Lesions (continued)

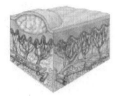

Tumor—Elevated solid, diameter more than 2 cm, may be same color as skin

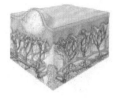

Pustule—Elevated area, diameter less than 1 cm, contains purulent fluid

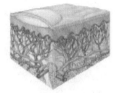

Vesicle—Elevated area, diameter less than 1 cm, contains serous fluid

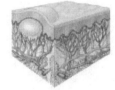

Cyst—Elevated, palpable area containing liquid or viscous matter

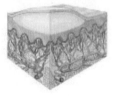

Bulla—Vesicle with diameter more than 1 cm

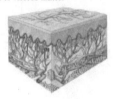

Telangiectasia—Red, threadlike line

Secondary Lesions

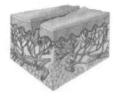

Fissure—Linear red crack ranging into dermis

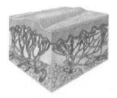

Scar—Fibrous, depth varies, color ranges from white to red

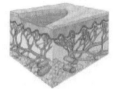

Erosion—Depression in epidermis, caused by tissue loss

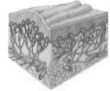

Keloid—Elevated scar, irregular shape, larger than original wound

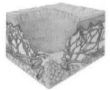

Ulcer—Red or purplish depression ranging into dermis, caused by tissue loss

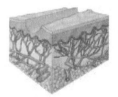

Excoriation—Linear, may be hollow or crusted, caused by loss of epidermis leaving dermis exposed

THE PHYSICAL EXAM

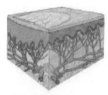

Scale—Elevated area of excessive exfoliation, varies in thickness, shape, and dryness, and ranges in color from white to silver or tan

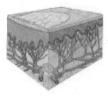

Lichenification—Thickening and hardening of epidermis with emphasized lines in skin, resembles lichen

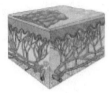

Crust—Reddish, brown, black, tan, or yellowish dried blood, serum, or pus

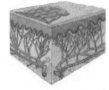

Atrophy—Skin surface thins and markings disappear, semitransparent parchment-like appearance

THE HAIR

Exam

Inspect and palpate the hair and scalp, noting the color, quality, distribution, quantity, and texture.

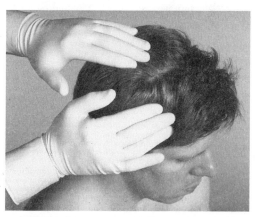

Normal

Clean scalp with no scaling, lesions, redness, lumps, or tenderness.

Abnormal

Finding	Significance
Generalized hair loss	Chemotherapy
Hirsuitism	Hormonal imbalance
Mild flaking	Dandruff
Heavy scaling	Psoriasis
Greasy scaling	Seborrheic dermatitis

THE NAILS

Exam

Inspect and palpate the fingernails and toenails for color beneath the transparent nail, ridging, grooves, depressions, and pitting. Gently squeeze the nail between your thumb and forefinger to test for adherence to the nail bed.

Normal

Pink color in caucasians and black and brown in blacks. No ridges, grooves, depressions, or pitting.

Abnormal

Condition	Description
Clubbing	Clubbing occurs when normal connective tissue and capillaries increase the angle between the plate and proximal nail to greater than 180 degrees. The distal phalanx of each finger is rounded and bulbous. The proximal nail feels spongy. This is caused by the chronic hypoxia found in cardiopulmonary diseases and lung cancer.
Paronychia	This is an inflammation of the proximal and lateral nail folds. It may be acute or chronic. The folds appear red and swollen, and tender. The cuticle may not be visible. People who frequently immerse their hands in water are susceptible.
Onycholysis	The nail bed separates from the nail plate. It begins distally and enlarges the free edge of the nail. There are many causes, including hyperthyroidism.
Terry's nails	These appear as a mostly whitish nail with a band of reddish-brown at the distal nail tip. This may be seen in aging and with people suffering from liver cirrhosis, congestive heart failure, and diabetes.
White spots	Trauma to the nail often results in white spots that grow out with the nail. They often follow the curvature of the cuticle and can be the result of overzealous manicuring.
Transverse white lines	These are lines that parallel the lunula, rather than the cuticle. They may appear following a severe illness. They appear from under the proximal nail folds and grow out with the nail.
Psoriasis	These appear as small pits in the nails and may be an early sign of psoriasis.
Beau's lines	These are transverse depressions in the nails and are associated with severe illness. As with the Transverse white lines, they form under the nail fold and grow out with the nail. You may be able to estimate the timing or length of an illness by the location of the line.

Exam

Inspect and palpate the head for the general size and contour of the skull, tenderness, deformities (depressions or protrusions), and areas of unusual warmth.

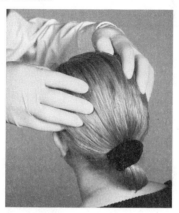

Normal

Symmetrical and smooth cranium.

Abnormal

Finding	Significance
Depression	Depressed skull fracture
Warmth/wetness	Scalp laceration
Protrusion	Skull fracture, impaled object, lesion

Exam

Inspect and palpate the face for symmetry, involuntary movements, masses, edema, periorbital ecchymosis (Raccoon's eyes), mastoid discoloration (Battle's sign), and facial bone stability.

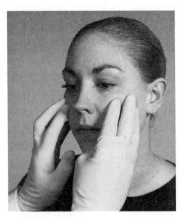

Normal

Symmetrical and stable facial bones

Abnormal

Finding	Significance
Asymmetry	Stroke, Bell's palsy, trauma
Periorbital ecchymosis	Basilar skull fracture, orbital fracture
Battle's sign	Basilar skull fracture
Facial instability	Fracture

THE TEMPOROMANDIBULAR JOINT

Exam

Ask your patient to open his mouth as you palpate TMJ for tenderness, swelling, and range of motion.

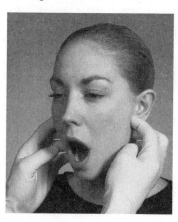

Normal

The tips of your fingers should drop into the joint space.

Abnormal

Tenderness, swelling, or pain during range of motion exam all suggest a TMJ abnormality.

THE EXTERNAL EYE

Exam

Examine the external structure of the eyes for symmetry in size, shape, and contour, the position of the eyelids in relation to the eyeballs, and complete closure. Examine the sclera and conjunctiva for color, swelling, nodules, and discharge.

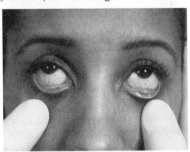

Normal

Equal size, shape, and contour. The lids should cover the upper quarter of the iris and close completely. The conjunctiva should be clear and transparent. The sclera should be white.

Abnormal

Finding	Significance
Droopy eyelid (ptosis)	Muscle weakness, CN-III nerve damage, sympathic interruption
Pale eyelid	Shock, anemia
Cyanotic eyelid	Hypoxia
Redness	Allergies, infection
Red spot	Hemorrhage
Yellow sclera	Liver disease
Yellow discharge	Infection
Clear discharge	Allergies
Periorbital edema	Allergies, inflammation, crying

Exam

Test for visual acuity with a wall chart (from 20 feet) or visual acuity card (from 14 inches) and read the number corresponding to the smallest line your patient can read.

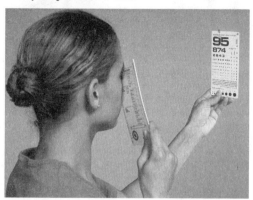

Normal

20/20

Abnormal

Anything greater than 20/20

THE PHYSICAL EXAM

84	✈	20/800
59	✈ ✈	20/400
7 3 6 2	✈ ✈ ✈	20/200
8 2 4 6 7	✈ ✈ ✈	20/100
6 7 5 3 9 4	✈ ✈ ✈	20/70
2 6 4 8 5 3	✈ ✈ ✈	20/50
5 7 8 3 6 9	✈ ✈ ✈	20/40
8 3 2 5 9 4	✈ ✈ ✈	20/30
3 4 5 7 6 8	✈ ✈ ✈	20/25

Hold this page 14 inches from eye.

VISUAL FIELDS

Exam

Test the visual fields by confrontation. Sit directly in front of your patient. Have him cover his left eye while you cover your right eye. Ask him to look at your nose. Hold a brightly colored object in your left hand and extend your left arm to the side. Slowly move your hand into his line of vision and have him tell you when he first sees it. Use your own peripheral vision as baseline normal from which to evaluate his. Now repeat the test from the other side, from above, and from below. Then perform the same test on the other eye.

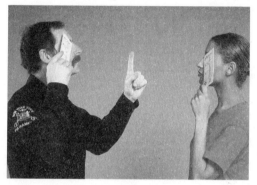

Normal

Normal vision in all fields

Abnormal

Visual Field Abnormalities

○	◑	Horizontal defect
○	●	Blind eye
◐	◑	Bitemporal hemianopsia
◑	◑	Homonymous hemianopsia
◕	◕	Homonymous quadrantic defect

Left   Right

Exam

Check your patient's pupil size and shape.

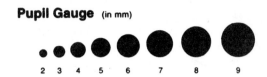

Pupil Gauge (in mm)

2 3 4 5 6 7 8 9

Direct Response

Shine a light into each eye and observe the reaction to the light in the same eye (direct response). It should constrict to light.

Consensual Response

Shine a light into each eye and observe the reaction in the opposite eye (consensual response). Both eyes should react simultaneously to the light.

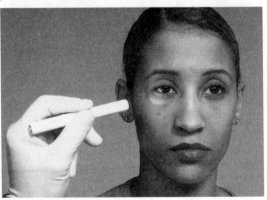

Near Response

Have your patient focus on an object somewhere in the distance. Then, ask him to focus on an object right in front of him. As he focuses on the near object, his pupils should constrict (near response).

Accommodation

Have your patient follow your finger as you move it from a distance to the bridge of the nose. The eyes should converge on the object as the pupils constrict (accommodation).

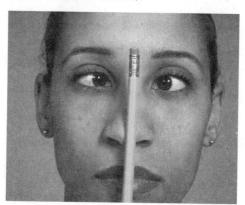

Normal

The pupils should be round and of equal size. They should constrict simultaneously to light and when focusing on near objects. The eyes should converge on an object as the pupils constrict.

Abnormal

Finding	Significance
Bilateral sluggishness	Global brain hypoxia, drug reaction
Constricted	Opiate overdose
Fixed, dilated	Brain death
Unequal	Increasing intracranial pressure, stroke

Exam

Have your patient follow your finger as you move it in an "H" pattern in front of him.

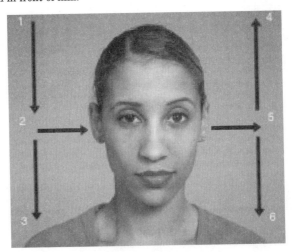

Normal

Normally the patient will move his eyes in conjugate (together) fashion to follow your finger.

Abnormal

He may exhibit a nystagmus, a fine jerking of the eyes at the far extremes of the test. Inability to move the eyes in any direction suggests a cranial nerve or extraocular muscle problem.

CORNEAL REFLEX

Exam

Touch the eye gently with a strand of cotton and watch for your patient to blink.

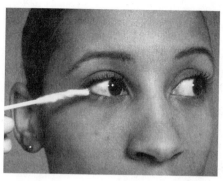

Normal

Your patient should blink.

Abnormal

No response to touch

Exam

Inspect and palpate the external ears and surrounding area for symmetry, size, shape, landmarks, color, positioning, deformities, lumps, skin lesions, tenderness, and erythema. Check the ear canal for drainage or excessive wax.

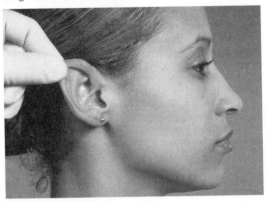

Normal

Symmetrical with no pain or tenderness

Abnormal

Finding	Significance
Pain/tenderness	Otitis, mastoiditis
Otorrhea	Ruptured eardrum, infection, skull fracture
Mastoid discoloration	Basilar skull fracture

HEARING ACUITY

Exam

Check for hearing acuity by having your patient occlude one ear. Test the other ear by whispering, then speaking, words toward the open ear. Then test the other ear in the same manner.

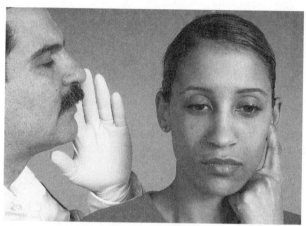

Normal

Equal, grossly normal hearing in both ears

Abnormal

Finding	Significance
Hearing loss, tinnitus	Trauma, wax, tympanic membrane rupture, drugs, surgery, loud noise exposure

THE NOSE

Exam

Inspect and palpate the external nose for symmetry in shape and color, depressions, deformities, and tenderness. Inspect the internal nose with an otoscope for deviations, perforations, and mucosal discharge (color, quantity, and consistency).

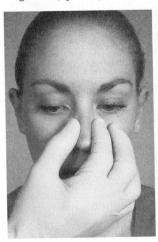
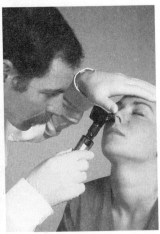

Test for obstruction of the discharge. Test for nasal obstruction by occluding one side of the nose and having your patient breathe through the other side.

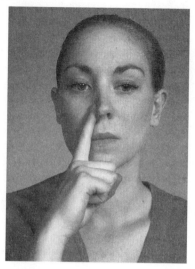

Normal

Symmetrical with no depressions, deformities, or tenderness. Some unilateral nasal obstruction is normal.

Abnormal

Finding	Significance
Nasal flaring	Respiratory distress
Watery rhinitis	Seasonal allergies
Purulent rhinitis	Infection
Epistaxis	Trauma, hypertension, septal defect
Excessive obstruction	Deviated septum, foreign body, secretions, edema, cocaine use

THE PARANASAL SINUSES

Exam

Inspect and palpate the frontal and maxillary sinuses for swelling and tenderness. Percuss the zygoma to elicit pain.

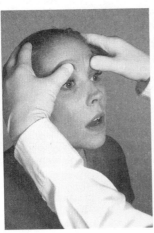 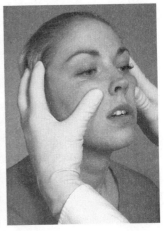

Normal

No pain or tenderness

Abnormal

Swelling or tenderness suggests a sinus infection or obstruction.

THE LIPS

Exam

Observe the condition and color of the lips. Note any lesions, swelling, lumps, cracks, or scaliness. Gently palpate the lips with the jaw closed and note any lesions, nodules, or fissures especially at the corners. Observe the undersurface of the upper and lower lip.

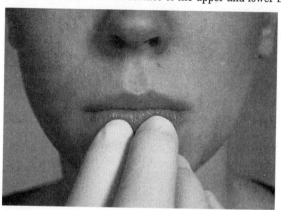

Normal

Pink, smooth, and symmetrical and devoid of lesions, swelling, lumps, cracks, or scaliness

Abnormal

Finding	Significance
Dry, cracked	Wind damage, dehydration
Swelling	Infection
Edema	Allergic reaction
Lesions	Infection, irritation, skin cancer
Pallor	Shock, anemia
Cyanosis	Respiratory or cardiac insufficiency

Exam

With a tongue blade, examine the oral mucosa for color, ulcers, white patches, and nodules, including under the tongue. Inspect the teeth for color, shape, position, and for any missing or loose teeth.

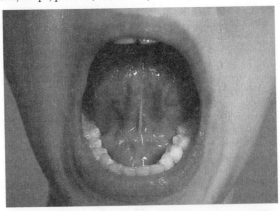

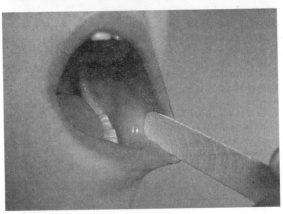

Press the tongue blade down on the middle third of the tongue and have your patient say "aaaaahhhh." Examine the posterior pharynx, the palatine tonsils, and the movement of the uvula. Inspect the tonsils for color and symmetry. Look for exudate, pus, ulcers, or swelling. Note any odors coming from your patient's mouth.

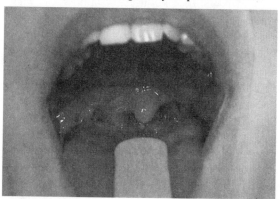

Normal

Pink mucosa, symmetrical structures, no exudate, ulcers or swelling. No unusual odors. The uvula should move straight up with no deviation.

Abnormal

Finding	Significance
Swollen, bleeding gums	Periodontal disease
Redness, exudate	Infection
Coffee grounds	Upper GI bleed
Fecal odor	Bowel obstruction
Acidic smell	Stomach contents
Acetone odor	Diabetic ketoacidosis
Pink-tinged sputum	Acute pulmonary edema
Cloudy, yellow phlegm	Respiratory infection

Exam

Inspect the neck for general symmetry, visible masses, obvious deformity, deviation, tugging, surgical scars, gland enlargement, and visible lymph nodes. Look for jugular vein distention while your patient is sitting up, and at a 45° incline. Palpate the trachea for midline position.

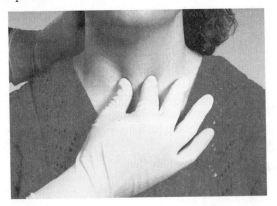

Normal

Symmetry with no visible masses. Trachea is midline with no signs of lateral movement or displacement. No JVD at 45°.

Abnormal

Finding	Significance
Visible midline mass	Goiter (enlarged thyroid)
Deviated trachea	Tension pneumothorax (late)
Tracheal tugging	Pneumothorax, respiratory distress
JVD	Right heart failure, tension pneumothorax, cardiac tamponade, pulmonary embolism
Subcutaneous emphysema	Laryngotracheal tear, pneumothorax
Neck muscle use	Difficulty in inspiration

THE THYROID GLAND

Exam

Palpate the thyroid gland from behind your patient. Rest your thumbs on his trapezius muscles and place two fingers of each hand on the sides of the trachea just beneath the cricoid cartilage. Have your patient swallow and feel for the movement of the gland.

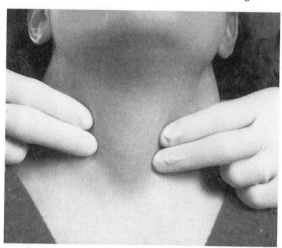

Normal
Small, smooth, and free of nodules

Abnormal
Any enlargement or nodules

THE LYMPH NODES

Exam
Using the pads of your fingers, palpate the nodes by moving the skin over the underlying tissues in each area. When swollen, the nodes are palpable, sometimes even visible. Note their size, shape, mobility, consistency, and tenderness.

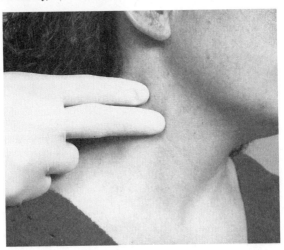

Normal
The nodes are not visible nor palpable when healthy.

Abnormal

Finding	Significance
Tender, swollen, and mobile nodes	Inflammation from infection
Hard or fixed nodes	Malignancy

THE CHEST—INSPECTION

Exam

Inspect the anterior and posterior chest wall and assess its symmetry. Do both sides of his chest wall rise in unison? Note accessory muscle use, retractions, floating segments, open wounds, anterior–posterior diameter.

Normal

The normal chest is symmetrical, with no exaggerated muscle use or retractions. The chest wall is wider than it is deep.

Abnormal

Finding	Significance
Funnel chest	The lower portion of the sternum is depressed.
Pigeon chest	The sternum caves outward.
Barrel chest	Equal anterior-posterior to transverse diameters
Retractions	Difficulty inhaling
Floating segment	Flail segment—trauma

THE PHYSICAL EXAM

Exam

Palpate the rib cage for rigidity. Feel for tenderness, deformities, depressions, loose segments, asymmetry, and crepitus. Evaluate for equal expansion. Lightly grasp his lateral rib cage with your spread hands. Ask him to inhale deeply and watch as your thumbs separate symmetrically as he inhales.

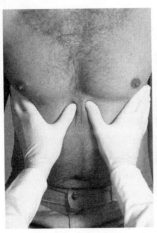 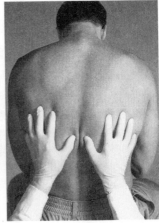

Normal

Normally the separation will increase by 3–5 centimeters during deep inspiration.

Abnormal

If you detect decreased thoracic expansion, or feel unilateral delay, suspect a disorder of the underlying lung, pleura, or diaphragm.

Exam

Place the palm of your hand on your patient's chest wall and have him say "ninety-nine" or "one-on-one." As he does, palpate the posterior chest, feel the vibrations in different areas of the chest wall, and compare symmetrical areas of the lungs. Identify and note any areas of increased, decreased, or absent vibrations.

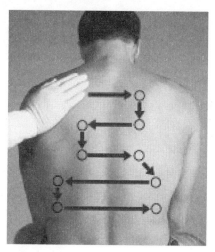

Normal

Normal vibration is constant in all areas of the lungs.

Abnormal

Finding	Significance
Increased vibrations	Tumor, pneumonia, or pulmonary fibrosis
Decreased vibrations	Pleural effusion, emphysema, pneumothorax

Exam

Percuss the chest symmetrically from the apices to the bases at
5-centimeter intervals, avoiding bony areas. Percuss at least twice
in each area and compare both sides of the thorax. Identify and note
any area of abnormal percussion.

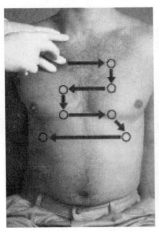 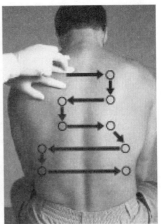

Normal

Sound	Description	Location
Tympany	Drumlike	Stomach
Hyperresonance	Booming	Hyperinflated lung
Resonance	Hollow	Normal lung
Dull	Thud	Solid organs
Flat	Extremely dull	Muscle, atelectasis

Abnormal

Finding	Significance
Bilateral hyperresonance	Asthma, COPD
Unilateral hyperresonance	Pneumothorax
Unilaterally dull	Hemothorax, pneumonia

Exam

Auscultate all lung fields and compare side-to-side. Evaluate the normal breath sounds produced by airflow through the upper and lower airways.

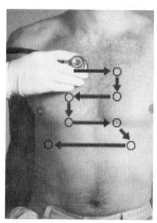 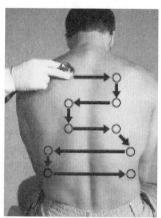

Normal

There should be bilateral equality and adequacy of air movement and no adventitious sounds.

Abnormal

Finding	Significance
Bilateral crackles	Left heart failure, bronchitis, interstitial lung disease
Localized crackles	Pneumonia, embolism
Diffuse wheezes	Asthma, emphysema, CHF
Local wheezes	Pneumonia, foreign body aspiration
Bilateral rhonchi	Bronchitis
Localized rhonchi	Pneumonia
Stridor	Laryngotracheal obstruction
Pleural rub	Pneumonia, pleurisy

TRANSMITTED VOICE SOUNDS

Exam

Ask the patient to say the following while you auscultate the chest:

"Ninety-nine" (Bronchophony)

Whisper "ninety-nine" (Whispered pectoriloquoy)

"E" (Egophony)

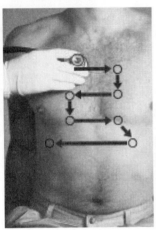 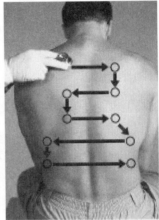

Normal

You should hear muffled, nondistinct sounds. For egophony, you should hear a muffled, long "E."

Abnormal

If you hear these words clearly, or if the "E" changes to "A," suspect that fluid (water, blood) or consolidated tissue (pus, tumor) has replaced the normally air-filled lung.

CARDIOVASCULAR

Exam

Reassess the carotid pulse, noting its rate, quality, and regularity. Compare it to earlier findings. Auscultate for carotid bruits.

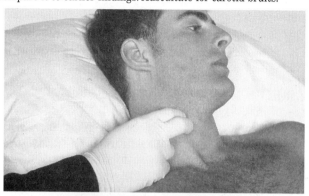

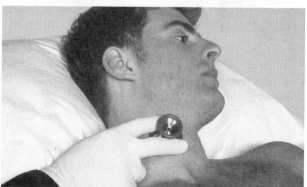

Normal

Equal, strong, regular carotid pulse with rate within normal limits for age and condition. No carotid bruits.

Abnormal

See earlier for pulse abnormalities. Carotid bruits suggest obstruction.

THE PHYSICAL EXAM

Exam

Position your patient supine with the head elevated to about 30°.

Turning his head away from the side you are assessing, identify the external jugular veins on both sides and locate the pulsations of the internal jugular veins. Look for the pulsation in the area around the suprasternal notch and where the sternocleidomastoid muscle inserts on the clavicle and manubrium. Identify the internal jugular vein's highest point of pulsation and measure its vertical distance to the sternal angle (midline at the 2nd costal cartilage). To do this, place the ruler perpendicular to the chest at the sternal angle and position a straightedge at a right angle to the ruler. Lower the straightedge until it rests atop the jugular vein pulsation. The corresponding ruler mark is your measurement. Examine the external jugular veins for equality and distention.

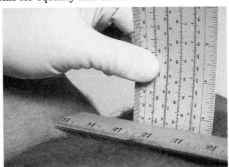

Normal

Normal venous pressure is 1–2 cm. If you cannot visualize the pulsations, observe the point where the external jugular veins collapse and use the same measuring parameters.

Abnormal

Abnormal bilateral distention indicates that something is blocking venous return to the heart (e.g., congestive heart failure, cardiac tamponade, etc.) or fluid volume overload. Unilateral distention suggests a localized problem.

THE POINT OF MAXIMUM IMPULSE (PMI)

Exam

Have your patient lie comfortably with his head raised about 30°. Inspect and palpate the chest for the PMI. First, look for a pulsation at the cardiac apex. The pulsation you will look for represents the apical impulse, or PMI. If you cannot see it at first, ask your patient to exhale and stop breathing for a few seconds. Look for it again and note its location. Percussion may be helpful if you are having a difficult time palpating the PMI. Start laterally and work your way toward the midline. When you hear a change from resonance (lung) to dull (heart), you have located the PMI.

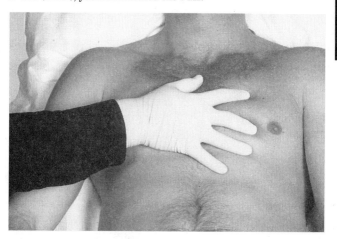

Normal

The PMI is normally found at the 5th intercostal space, just medial to the mid-clavicular line.

Abnormal

Lateral displacement of the PMI suggests an enlarged right ventricle or right-sided tension pneumothorax. The PMI may be displaced upward and to the left in pregnant women.

Exam

Using the diaphragm of your stethoscope, auscultate your patient's anterior chest for normal heart sounds and abnormal or extra heart sounds. Listen for S_1 at the 5th intercostal space at the left sternal border (tricuspid valve) and at the PMI (mitral valve), using the diaphragm of your stethoscope. Listen for S_2 at the 2nd intercostal space at the right sternal border (aortic valve) and 2nd intercostal space at the left sternal border (pulmonic valve), using the diaphragm of your stethoscope.

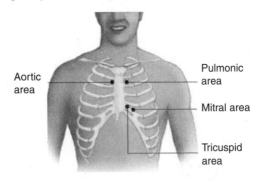

Normal

The normal heart sounds are S_1 and S_2, also known as the "lub-dub." There should be no other sounds.

Abnormal

Finding	Significance
S_3 ("lub-dub-dee")	Ventricular overload or failure
S_4 ("dee-lub-dub")	Decreased ventricular compliance
Ejection click	A stiff or stuck valve
Opening snap	Valve stenosis
Friction rub	Inflammation
Murmur	Turbulent blood flow

THE ABDOMEN—INSPECTION

Exam

Inspect the skin of the abdomen and flanks for scars, dilated veins, stretch marks, rashes, lesions, and pigmentation changes. Assess the size and shape of the abdomen. Note its symmetry. Check for bulges, hernias, or distended flanks. Now look at his umbilicus. Note its location and contour and observe for any signs of herniation or inflammation. Check for any visible pulsation, peristalsis, or masses.

Normal

The normal abdomen is scaphoid (concave), flat, or round. You may see the normal pulsation of the aorta just lateral to the umbilicus. There should be no distention, bulging, or exaggerated pulsation.

Abnormal

Finding	Significance
Distention	Air, fluid in the stomach
Cullen's sign	Intraabdominal bleeding
Grey-Turner's sign	Intraabdominal bleeding
Ascites	Congestive heart failure
Suprapubic bulge	Distended bladder or pregnant uterus
Inguinal bulge	Hernia
Femoral bulge	Hernia
Exaggerated pulsation	Aortic aneurysm
Visible peristalsis	Bowel obstruction

Exam

Auscultate for bowel sounds, and other sounds such as bruits, throughout the abdomen, noting their location, frequency, and character. Listen for at least 2 minutes if the abdomen is silent.

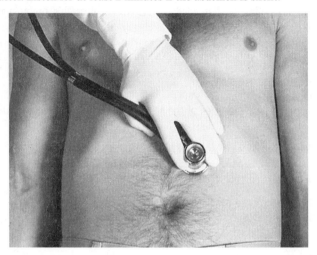

Normal

Normal bowel sounds consist of a variety of high-pitched gurgles and clicks that occur every 5–15 seconds.

Abnormal

Finding	Significance
Increased sounds	Diarrhea or intestinal obstruction
Decreased sounds	Paralytic ileus or peritonitis
Bruits	Abdominal aortic aneurysm or renal artery stenosis

THE ABDOMEN—PERCUSSION

Exam

Percuss the abdomen in the same sequence you used for auscultation; note the distribution of tympany and dullness.

Normal

Expect to hear tympany in most of the abdomen. Expect to hear dullness over the solid abdominal organs such as the liver and spleen.

Abnormal

Finding	Significance
Large, dull mass	Large liver or spleen, pregnant uterus, ovarian tumor, distended bladder
Dullness in flanks	Ascites
Tympanic throughout abdomen	Intestinal obstruction

Exam

Ask your patient if he has any pain or tenderness. If he does, palpate that area last using gentle pressure with a single finger. Perform light palpation by moving your hand slowly and just lifting it off the skin. Watch your patient's face for signs of discomfort. Identify any masses and note their size, location, contour, tenderness, pulsations, and mobility.

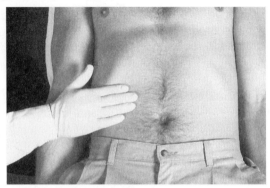

Perform deep palpation to detect large masses or tenderness. Use one hand on top of another and push down slowly, and then release your hand quickly off the tender area (rebound tenderness).

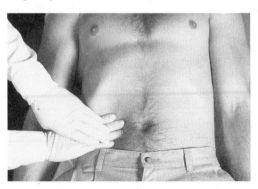

To test for fluid wave, ask your partner to press the edge of his hand firmly down the midline of the abdomen. Tap one flank with your fingertips and feel for the impulse's transmission to the other flank through excess fluid.

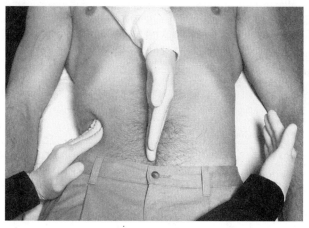

Normal
The normal abdomen is soft and nontender.

Abnormal

Finding	Significance
Pain upon light palpation or cough	Peritonitis
Rebound tenderness	Peritonitis
Involuntary rigidity	Peritonitis
Ascites	Congestive heart failure, renal failure

THE FEMALE GENITALIA

Exam

Look at the mons pubis, labia, and perineum for abnormalities such as inflammation or lesions. Check the bases of pubic hair for signs of lice such as excoriation, or small, itchy, red maculopapules. Now retract the outer labia and inspect the inner labia and urethral meatus (opening). Assess for vaginal discharge.

Normal

The normal vaginal discharge is clear or cloudy and has little or no odor.

Abnormal

Finding	Significance
Lesions	Sebaceous cyst or STD (syphilis or herpes simplex)
White discharge	Candidiasis, fungal infection
Yellow, green, discharge	Bacterial infection (gonorrhea)

THE MALE GENITALIA

Exam

Inspect the skin around the base of the penis for abnormalities such as lesions that may be caused by sexually transmitted diseases. Also check the bases of pubic hair for signs of lice such as excoriation, or small, itchy, red maculopapules. Next inspect the glans for signs of degeneration or other abnormalities. If the foreskin is present, ask your patient to retract it. Note any abnormalities and the location of the urethral meatus and assess any discharge. Inspect the anterior surface of the scrotum and note its contour. Then, lift the scrotum to inspect its posterior surface and note any swelling or lumps.

Normal

There should be no lesions or deformities. Normally no discharge is present.

Abnormal

Finding	Significance
Scrotal swelling	Acute epididymitis or testicular torsion
Profuse, yellow discharge	Gonorrhea
Scant, clear or white discharge	Nongonococcal urethritis

THE ANUS

Exam
Place your patient on his left side with his legs flexed and his buttocks near the edge of the examination table. Glove your hands and spread the buttocks apart. Inspect the sacrococcygeal and perianal areas. Palpate any abnormal areas carefully and note any tenderness or inflammation.

Normal
The sacrococcygeal and perianal areas should be free of lumps, ulcers, inflammations, rashes, or excoriation.

Abnormal
Lumps, ulcers, inflammations, rashes, or excoriation.

THE JOINTS

Exam
Perform the following five tests on all joints:

1. Inspect the joint.
2. Palpate the joint.
3. Passive range of motion (ROM)
4. Active range of motion
5. Active range of motion against resistance

Normal
The joints should be symmetrical with free movement in the normal range of motion. Passive and active range should be equal.

Abnormal

Finding	Significance
Swelling	Trauma
Subcutaneous nodules	Rheumatoid arthritis or rheumatic fever
Skin redness	Inflammation or arthritis
Deformities	Misalignment of the articulating bones, dislocation, or subluxation
Asymmetry	Rheumatoid arthritis
Hot area	Arthritis
Difficulty with ROM	Joint problem
Difficulty with active only	Weakened muscle or nerve disorder
Decreased ROM	Arthritis or injury
Increased ROM	Loosening of support structures
Crepitus	Inflamed joint or osteoarthritis

THE HANDS AND WRISTS

Exam

Inspect and palpate each of the following joints for swelling, sponginess, bony enlargement, or tenderness:

1. Distal interphalangeal (DIP)
2. Proximal interphalangeal (PIP)
3. Metacarpal-phalangeal (MCP)
4. Wrist

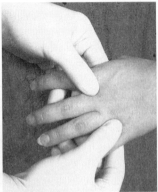

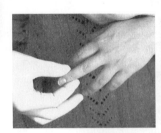

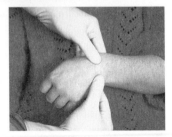

To assess range of motion, ask your patient to make a fist with each hand and then open his fist and extend and spread his fingers. He should be able to make a tight fist and spread his fingers smoothly and easily. Next ask him to flex, then extend his wrist.

Normal flexion is 90°, normal extension is 70°.

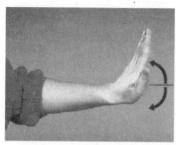

Extension

Neutral

Flexion

Check for radial and ulnar deviation by asking him to flex his wrist and move his hands medially and laterally. Normal ulnar deviation is 45°, normal radial deviation is 20°.

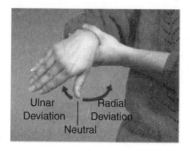

Ulnar
Deviation

Radial
Deviation

Neutral

If your patient complains of hand pain and numbness, especially at night, suspect carpal tunnel syndrome, the painful inflammation of the median nerve. To detect additional signs of this disorder, hold your patient's wrists in acute flexion for 60 seconds. In carpal tunnel syndrome, he will develop numbness or tingling to areas innervated by the median nerve (e.g., over the palmar surface of his thumb index and middle finger, and part of his ring finger).

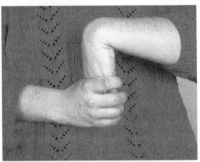

Abnormal

Throughout these maneuvers, watch for a decreased range of motion, deformities, redness, swelling, nodules, or muscular atrophy.

THE ELBOWS

Exam

To examine the elbow, support your patient's forearm so that his elbow is flexed about 70°. Inspect the elbow joint and note any deformities, swelling, or nodules. Palpate the joint structures for tenderness, swelling, or thickening. Inflammation of the medial (tennis elbow) and lateral (golfer's elbow) epicondyles suggests tendonitis at those muscle insertion sites.

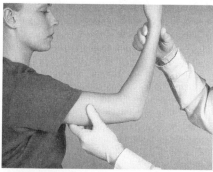

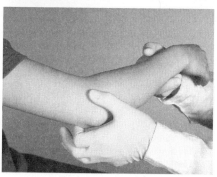

To assess range of motion, ask your patient to flex and extend his elbow.

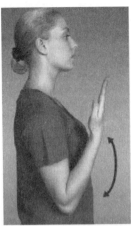

Then test for pronation and supination of the wrist. Have him flex his elbows and turn his palms up and down. Normal flexion is 160°; normal pronation and supination are 90°.

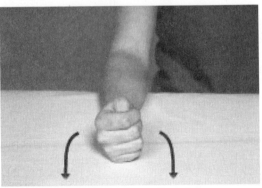

Supination   Pronation

THE SHOULDERS

Exam

To assess your patient's shoulders, look at them from the front and then look at his scapulae from the back. Inspect the entire shoulder girdle for swelling, deformities, or muscular atrophy. Before you palpate, ask him if he has any pain in the shoulders. If so, palpate this area last. Palpate the shoulders with your fingertips moving along the clavicles out toward the humerus. Palpate the sternoclavicular joint, acromioclavicular joint, subacromial region, and the bicipital groove for tenderness (biceps tendonitis) or swelling (bursitis). Now palpate over the greater tubercle of the humerus as you abduct the arm at the shoulder. Then, palpate the scapulae.

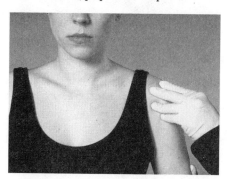

To assess range of motion, ask your patient to raise both arms forward and straight overhead (flexion). Next ask him to extend both arms behind his back (extension). Normal flexion is 180°; normal extension is 50°.

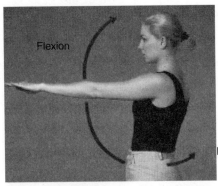

Flexion

Extension

Now have him raise both his arms overhead from the side (abduction). Then ask him to lower his arms and swing them as far as he can across his body (adduction). Normal abduction is 180°; normal adduction is 75°.

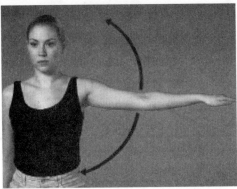

Abduction

Adduction

Finally, have him adduct his shoulders to 90°, pronate and flex his elbows 90° to the front of his body. Now ask him to rotate his shoulders to the "goal post" position" (external rotation). Then ask him to rotate his shoulders in the opposite direction so that his hands point down (internal rotation). Normal external and internal rotation is 90°.

External
Rotation

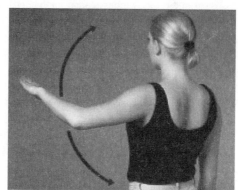

Internal
Rotation

Abnormal

Throughout these maneuvers, watch for a decreased range of motion, deformities, redness, swelling, nodules, or muscular atrophy.

Exam

Inspect the feet and ankles for obvious deformities, nodules, swelling, calluses, or corns. Palpate the anterior aspect of each ankle joint with your thumbs and note any sponginess, swelling, or tenderness. Feel along the Achilles tendon for tenderness or nodules. Exert pressure between your thumbs and fingers on each metatarsophalangeal joint. Acute inflammation of these joints suggests gout. Tenderness is an early sign of rheumatoid arthritis.

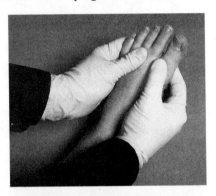

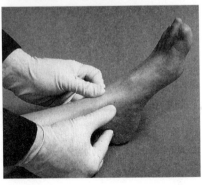

To test range of motion, ask your patient to bring his foot upward (dorsiflexion). Then have him point it downward (plantar flexion). Normal dorsiflexion is 20°; normal plantar flexion is 45°.

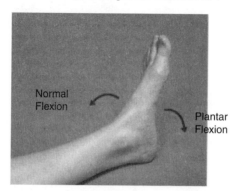

Normal Flexion

Plantar Flexion

Then, while stabilizing the ankle with one hand, grasp the heel with the other hand and invert the foot, then evert it. Normal inversion is 30° and normal eversion is 20°.

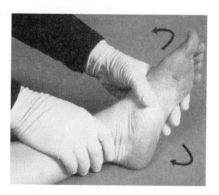

Finally, flex and extend the toes. Expect a great range of motion in these joints, especially the big toes.

Extension   Flexion

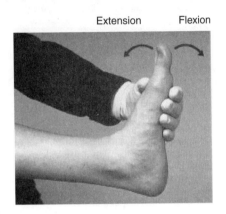

Abnormal

Throughout these maneuvers, watch for a decreased range of motion, deformities, redness, swelling, nodules, or muscular atrophy. Pain with dorsiflexion (Homans' sign) suggests a deep vein thrombosis (DVT).

THE KNEES

Exam

Inspect your patient's knees for alignment and deformities. Look for the concave areas that usually appear on each side of the patella and just above it. The loss of these areas indicates swelling in the knee or the surrounding structures. If swelling is present, milk the medial aspect of the knee firmly upward 2 or 3 times to displace the fluid. Then press the knee just behind the lateral margin of the patella and watch for a return of fluid (a positive sign for effusion). Feel for any thickening or swelling around the patella. Compress the patella and move it against the femur. Note any pain or tenderness.

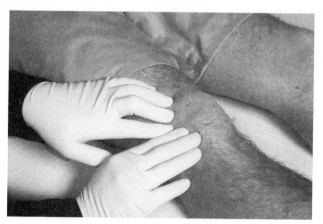

To test the joint, have your patient flex his knee to 90°. Press your thumbs into the joint and palpate along the tibial margins from the patellar tendon laterally. Palpate along the course of each ligament and note any points of tenderness. If your patient has tenderness, expect damage to the meniscus (cartilage) or lateral ligaments. If you feel irregular bony ridges, suspect osteoarthritis. Now test for stability of the medial and collateral ligaments by moving the knee joint from side to side. There should be little movement.

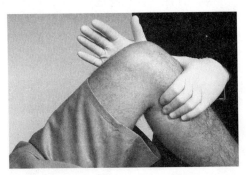

Evaluate the anterior and posterior cruciate ligaments by using the "drawer" test. Try to move the knee joint anterior and posterior, much like opening and closing a drawer. There should be little movement.

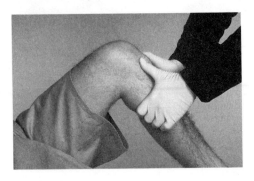

To test range of motion, have your patient sit at the edge of the exam table with his lower legs dangling. Ask him to extend his leg out. Now ask him to roll over and try to touch his foot to his back. Normal flexion is 135°, normal extension is 90°.

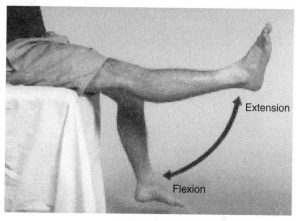

Abnormal

Throughout these maneuvers, watch for a decreased range of motion, deformities, redness, swelling, nodules, or muscular atrophy.

Exam

Inspect and palpate the hip for deformity, swelling, or sponginess. Palpate for tenderness all around the joint, including the three bursa and greater trochanter of the femur.

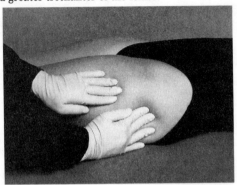

To test range of motion, with your patient supine, ask him to raise his knee to his chest and pull it firmly against his abdomen. Observe the degree of flexion at the knee and hip. Normal flexion is 120°.

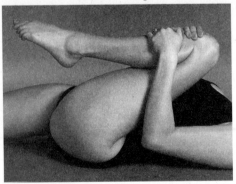

Now flex the hip at 90° and stabilize the thigh with one hand while you grasp the ankle with the other. Swing the lower leg medially to evaluate external rotation, and laterally to evaluate internal rotation. Arthritis restricts internal rotation. Normal external rotation is 45°; normal internal rotation is 40°.

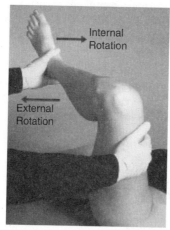

Test for hip abduction by first having your patient extend his legs. Then while you stabilize the anterior superior iliac spine with one hand, abduct the other leg until you feel the iliac spine move. This marks the degree of hip abduction. Normal abduction is 90°.

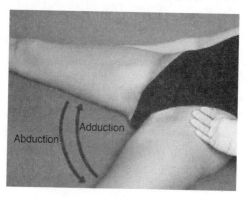

THE SPINE

Exam

Inspect your patient's head and neck for deformities, abnormal posture, and asymmetry of the skin folds. Ask him to bend forward slightly while you visually identify the spinous processes, the paravertebral muscles, the scapulae, the iliac crests, and the posterior iliac spines (usually marked by dimples). Draw imaginary horizontal lines across the shoulders and iliac crests. Now draw an imaginary vertical line down from T_1 to the space between the buttocks (gluteal cleft). Then observe him from the side. Evaluate the normal curves of the cervical, thoracic, and lumbar spine and note any irregularities.

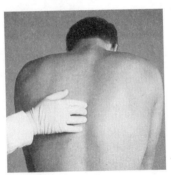

Normal

The head should be erect and the spine straight. The spine should be concave in cervical and lumbar regions, convex in thorax. No protrusions or visible spasms. Straight line from T_1 to the gluteal cleft. No deformity, tenderness or spasms on palpation.

Abnormal Spinal Curvatures

Condition	Description
Lordosis	Exaggerated lumbar concavity (swayback)
Kyphosis	Exaggerated thoracic concavity (hunchback)
Scoliosis	Lateral curvature

THE CERVICAL SPINE
Exam

First test for flexion by asking your patient to touch chin to chest. Next, ask him to bend his head backward. This tests extension.

Normal flexion is 45°; normal extension is 55°.

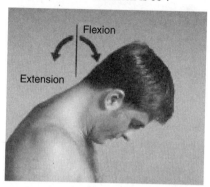

Now test for rotation by asking him to touch chin to each shoulder. Normal rotation is 70° to either side.

Rotation

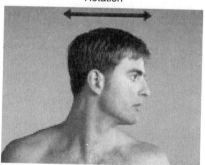

Finally, ask him to touch each ear to his shoulder without raising his shoulders. This assesses lateral bending. Normal lateral bending is 40° to either side.

Right   Left

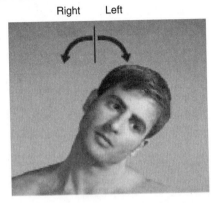

Abnormal

Any pain or tenderness during range of motion tests suggests a muscle spasm, ruptured ligament, or herniated disc. Decreased range of motion suggests a neurological or musculoskeletal dysfunction. Nuchal rigidity suggests meningitis.

THE LUMBAR SPINE
Exam

Test for flexion of the lower spine by asking your patient to bend and touch his toes. To assess extension, ask him to bend backward toward you. Note the smoothness and symmetry of the movement, the range of motion, and curves in the lumbar region. Observe the lumbar area during this exam. Normal flexion is 75–90°; normal extension is 30°.

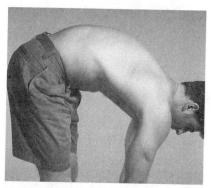

Then stabilize his pelvis with your hands and have him bend sideways (lateral bending). Normal lateral bending is 35° on either side.

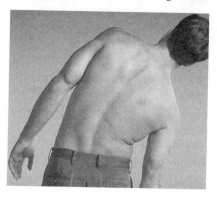

Finally, test spinal rotation by asking him to twist his shoulders one way, then the other. Normal rotation is 35° to either side.

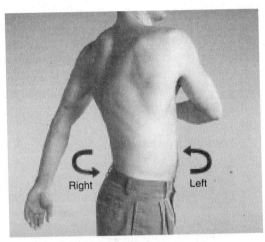

Right   Left

Abnormal

If the lumbar spine remains concave or appears asymmetrical during the range of motion tests, your patient may have a muscle spasm. If your patient complains of lower back pain radiating down the back of one leg, assess it by having him lie supine on the table. Ask him to raise his straightened leg until he feels pain. Note the elevation at which the pain occurs as well as the quality and distribution of the pain. Now dorsiflex your patient's foot and determine if this maneuver causes pain. Sharp pain that radiates from the back down the leg suggests compression of the nerve roots of the lower lumbar region. Now repeat this test with the other leg. Increased pain in the affected leg when the opposite leg is raised confirms the finding.

THE PERIPHERAL VASCULAR SYSTEM

Exam

Inspect all four extremities for size and symmetry. Evaluate the presence of swelling, venous congestion, the color of the skin and nail beds, and the skin texture.

Palpate the peripheral arteries to feel the pulsation of the blood flow, to assess skin temperature, and to check capillary refill. Note the rate, regularity, equality, and quality of the pulses on the scale below. Compare peripheral pulses bilaterally.

Score	Pulse Description
0	Absent
1+	Weak or thready
2+	Normal
3+	Bounding

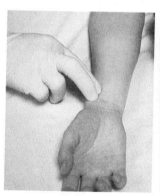 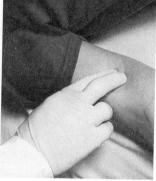

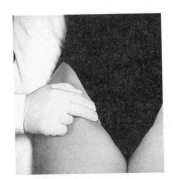

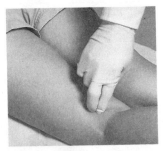

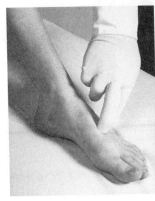

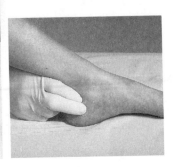

Palpate for pitting edema by pressing firmly with your thumb for five seconds over the top of the foot, behind each medial ankle, and over the shins. Pitting is a depression left by the pressure of your thumb. Normally there should be no depression.

Score	Pitting Depth
1+	1/4 inch or less
2+	1/4–1/2 inch
3+	1/4–1 inch
4+	1 inch or more

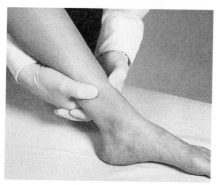

Abnormal

Finding	Significance
Unilateral weak or absent pulse	Arterial occlusion
Thrills	Cardiac murmur, vascular narrowing
Unilateral coldness	Arterial occlusion
Bilateral coldness	Environmental
Bilateral pitting edema	Congestive heart failure, renal failure
Unilateral pitting edema	DVT, venous occlusion
Yellow or brittle nails, poor color in fingertips	Chronic arterial insufficiency

THE NEUROLOGICAL EXAM

A comprehensive neurological exam includes the following components:

A. Mental Status and Speech
    1. Appearance and Behavior
    2. Speech and Language
    3. Mood
    4. Thought and Perceptions
    5. Insight and Judgment
    6. Memory and Attention

B. Cranial Nerves

C. Motor System
    1. General body structure
    2. Muscle bulk, tone, and strength
    3. Coordination

D. Sensory System
    1. Light touch
    2. Pain
    3. Temperature
    4. Position sense
    5. Vibration
    6. Discrimination

E. Reflexes
    1. Biceps
    2. Triceps
    3. Brachioradialis
    4. Quadriceps
    5. Achilles
    6. Abdominal
    7. Plantar

APPEARANCE AND BEHAVIOR

Exam

Is your patient alert and awake? Does he understand your questions? Does he respond appropriately and timely or does he drift off the topic easily or lose interest? If you detect an abnormality, continue with more specific questions. If your patient is awake and alert, observe his posture and motor behavior.

Normal

Your patient should be alert with eyes open and respond timely and appropriately to your questions. Unless he is in bed or on the ground, his posture should be erect.

Abnormal

Level of Response

Finding	Description
Lethargic	Drowsy, but will answer your questions appropriately and then fall asleep again.
Obtunded	Will open his eyes and look at you but respond slowly and confused.
Stuperous	Arousable for short periods of time but is not aware of his surroundings.
Comatose	In a state of profound unconsciousness and is totally unarousable.

Posture

Finding	Significance
Tense posture, restlessness, fidgeting	Anxiety
Crying, hand wringing, pacing	Agitated, depression
Hopeless, slumped posture, slowed movements	Depression
Singing, dancing, expansive movements	Manic

PERSONAL HYGIENE

Exam

Observe your patient's grooming and personal hygiene. How is he dressed? Note your patient's hair, teeth, nails, skin, and beard.

Normal

His clothes should be clean, pressed, and properly fastened. His appearance should be appropriate for the season, climate, and occasion. Hair, teeth, skin, nails should be well groomed.

Abnormal

A deterioration in grooming and personal hygiene in the previously well-groomed person may suggest an emotional problem, a psychiatric disorder, or organic brain disease. Patients with obsessive-compulsive behavior may exhibit excessive attention to their appearance. One-sided neglect may suggest a brain lesion.

FACIAL EXPRESSIONS

Exam

Observe his facial expressions.

Normal

Facial expressions should vary when talking with others and when the topic changes. Expressions should be appropriate. He should be able to express happiness, sadness, anger, depression.

Abnormal

Patients with Parkinson's disease have facial immobility. Patients with Bell's palsy or stroke may have unilateral immobility.

SPEECH AND LANGUAGE

Exam

Note the pattern of your patient's speech. Is your patient too talkative or silent? Does he speak spontaneously or only when you ask him a direct question?

Normal

Normally a person's speech has inflections, is clear and strong, fluent and articulate, and can increase in volume. There should be a clear expression of thoughts.

Abnormal

Finding	Significance
Slow, quiet speech	Depression
Fast, loud speech	Manic
Dysarthria (defective speech)	Motor deficit
Dysphonia (voice change)	Vocal cord problems
Aphasia (defective language)	Neurologic damage

MOOD

Exam

Observe your patient's mood from his verbal and nonverbal behavior. Note any mood swings or behaviors that suggest anxiety or depression.

Normal

Your patient's mood should be appropriate for his situation.

Abnormal

Is he sad, elated, angry, enraged, anxious, worried, detached, or indifferent? Assess the intensity of your patient's mood. How long has he been this way? Is he acting normally considering the circumstances? If your patient is depressed, is he suicidal? If you suspect the possibility of suicide, ask him directly about these feelings: "Have you ever thought of committing suicide?" If so, "Have you developed a plan?"

THOUGHTS

Exam

Assess how well your patient organizes his thoughts and speaks logically and coherently. Assess the thought content of your patient's responses.

Normal

Your patient should organize his thoughts and speak logically.

Abnormal

Finding	Possible Cause
Shifts between unrelated topics without realizing the thoughts are not connected.	Psychiatric disorders
Speaks constantly in related areas with no real conclusion or end-point.	Mania
Rambles with unrelated, illogical thoughts and disordered grammar.	Severe psychosis
Makes up facts or events.	Amnesia
Driven to perform to prevent some unrealistic future result.	Neurosis
Recurrent, uncontrollable fear of dread and doom.	Neurosis
Senses that things in the environment are strange or unreal.	Psychotic disorder
Has false, personal beliefs that are not shared by other members of the person's group.	Psychotic disorder

PERCEPTIONS

Exam

Figure out whether your patient perceives imaginary things. For example, he sees visions, hears voices, smells odors, and feels things that aren't there. Ask him about these false perceptions in the same way you would ask about anything else. For example: "When you see the pink elephants, what are they doing?"

Normal

Your patient should not perceive imaginary things, either by visual, audio, or tactile means.

Abnormal

Finding	Possible Cause
Misinterprets what is there (illusions).	Schizophrenia, post-traumatic stress disorders, and organic brain syndrome
Sees things that are not there (hallucinations).	Schizophrenia, post-traumatic stress disorders, and organic brain syndrome
Auditory and visual hallucinations	Psychedelic drug ingestion
Tactile hallucinations	Alcohol withdrawal

THE NEUROLOGICAL EXAM

INSIGHT AND JUDGMENT

Exam

Does he understand what is happening to him? Does he realize that what he thinks and how he feels are part of the illness? Patients with psychotic disorders may not have insight into their illness. Does your mature patient respond appropriately to questions concerning his family and personal life? Ask him what he would do if he cut himself shaving.

Normal

Your patient can evaluate the data and provide an adequate response.

Abnormal

Impaired judgment is common with emotional problems, mental retardation, and organic brain syndrome.

THE NEUROLOGICAL EXAM

ORIENTATION

Exam

Determine your patient's orientation. Does he know his name? Does he know the time of day, day of the week, month, season, and year? Does he know where he is, where he lives, the name of the city and state?

Normal

Your patient should be oriented to person, time, and place and respond appropriately to your questions.

Abnormal

Finding	Significance
Person disorientation	Trauma, seizures, amnesia
Time disorientation	Anxiety, depression, organic brain syndrome
Place disorientation	Psychiatric disorder, organic brain syndrome

CONCENTRATION

Exam

Assess your patient's ability to concentrate with the following three exercises:

Digit span   Have him repeat a series of numbers back to you.

Serial sevens   Ask him to start from 100 and subtract seven each time.

Backward spelling Ask your patient to spell a common five-letter word backward.

Normal

A person should be able to perform these tests without difficulty.

Abnormal

Poor performance could suggest delirium, dementia, mental retardation, loss of calculating ability, anxiety, depression, or alcohol intoxication.

THE NEUROLOGICAL EXAM

MEMORY

Exam

Assess your patient's memory with the following three exercises:

Immediate memory	Ask him to repeat three or four words that have no correlation such as "desk, toothbrush, six, and blue."
Recent memory	Ask him what he had for lunch or to repeat something he told you earlier in the interview.
Remote memory	Ask him about facts such as his wife's name, his son's birthday, or his Social Security number.

Normal

Your patient should be able to recall in all three categories without difficulty.

Abnormal

Long-term and short-term memory problems may be due to amnesia, anxiety, or organic causes.

THE CRANIAL NERVES

	Cranial Nerve	Function	Innervation
I	Olfactory	Sensory	Sense of smell
II	Optic	Sensory	Vision
III	Oculomotor	Motor	Eye movement
IV	Trochlear	Motor	Eye movement
V	Trigeminal	Both	Sensory to face, motor to chewing
VI	Abducens	Motor	Eye movement
VII	Facial	Both	Facial muscles
VIII	Acoustic	Sensory	Hearing and balance
IX	Glosso-pharyngeal	Both	Taste and gag reflex
X	Vagus	Both	Gag reflex and parasympathetic tone
XI	Accessory	Motor	Trapezius and sternocleido-mastoid muscles
XII	Hypoglossal	Motor	Tongue

The One-Minute Cranial Nerve Exam

Nerves	Test
II, III	Check direct pupillary response to light.
III, IV, VI	Do the "H" test for extraocular movement.
V	Clench teeth and palpate massiter muscles. Sensory to forehead, cheek, and chin.
VII	Smile wide and show teeth.
IX, X	Say "aaaaah," watch uvula. Gag reflex.
XI	Shrug shoulders/turn head against resistance.
VIII	Romberg test and hearing.

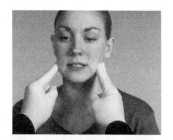

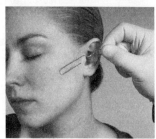

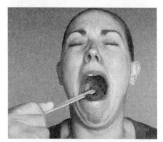

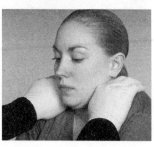

MOTOR SYSTEM

GENERAL BODY STRUCTURE

Exam

Inspect your patient's general body structure. What is his position at rest? Note any obvious asymmetries, deformities, or involuntary movements. Are there tremors, tics, or fasiculations (twitches)? If present, note their location, rate, quality, rhythm, amplitude, and how they relate to your patient's posture, activity, fatigue, emotion, and other factors. To assess involuntary movement, observe your patient throughout the exam.

Normal

Your patient should be erect and symmetrical with no involuntary movements or deformities.

Abnormal

Finding	Significance
Slumped to one side	Unilateral weakness or paralysis from trauma or stroke
Hand tremors during voluntary movement	Postural tremor
Hand tremor at rest, disappears during voluntary movement	Parkinson's disease

MUSCLE BULK

Exam

Evaluate your patient's muscle bulk, tone, and strength during passive and active range of motion tests.

Normal

Your patient should have normal muscle size in relation to his strength and exhibit no abnormal movements during range of motion tests.

Abnormal

Finding	Description
Atrophy	Decrease in bulk and strength
Hypertrophy	Increase in bulk and strength
Pseudohypertrophy	Increase in bulk, decrease in strength

MUSCLE TONE

Exam

Evaluate your patient's muscle tone during passive range of motion tests.

Normal

Your patient should exhibit normal muscle tone with fluid motion during test.

Abnormal

Finding	Description
Spasticity	Increased tone when passive movement is applied, especially at the end of range. Common in stroke.
Rigidity	Increased rigidity throughout movement (lead-pipe). Common in Parkinson's disease and extra-pyramidal reactions. Cog-wheel motion is a patient-applied resistance.
Flaccidity	Loss of muscle tone causing limb to be loose. Common in stroke, spinal cord lesion, and Guillian-Barre syndrome.
Paratonia	Sudden changes in tone with passive movement. Can be increased or decreased resistance. Common in dementia.

THE NEUROLOGICAL EXAM

MUSCLE STRENGTH
Exam
Evaluate your patient's muscle strength with passive and active range of motion tests for all muscle groups.

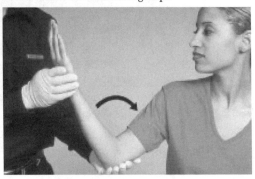

Normal
Your patient should exhibit bilaterally equal muscle strength during active range of motion tests against resistance.

Abnormal

Score	Description
5	Active movement against full resistance with no fatigue
4	Active movement against some resistance and gravity
3	Active movement against gravity
2	Active movement with gravity eliminated
1	Barely palpable muscle contraction with no movement
0	No visible or palpable muscle contraction

GAIT AND COORDINATION

Exam

To assess position sense and coordination, first assess your patient's gait. Ask him to walk across the room, turn, and come back. Now ask him to walk heel-to-toe in a straight line. This is known as tandem walking and may reveal an ataxia not previously seen. Now ask your patient to walk first on his toes, then on his heels. This will assess plantar flexion and dorsiflexion of the ankle as well as his balance. Next, ask him to hop in place on each foot in turn. Now ask him to do a shallow knee bend on each leg in turn.

Normal

Normally your patient will be able to maintain his balance, swing his arms at his side, and turn easily. He should also perform all of the above maneuvers easily and without problems. You may have to make reasonable modifications for an elderly patient.

Abnormal

If his gait is uncoordinated, reeling, or unstable, known as an ataxic gait, suspect cerebellar disease, loss of position sense, or intoxication. Difficulty in hopping may be the result of leg muscle weakness, lack of position sense, or cerebellar dysfunction. Difficulty doing shallow knee bends suggests muscle weakness in the pelvic girdle and legs.

THE NEUROLOGICAL EXAM

ROMBERG TEST/PRONATOR DRIFT

Exam

Next perform the Romberg test. Ask him to stand with his feet together and eyes open. Now have him close his eyes for 20 to 30 seconds. Observe his ability to maintain an upright position with minimal swaying and no support. Then check for pronator drift. Ask him to place his arms straight in front of him with his palms upright for 20–30 seconds.

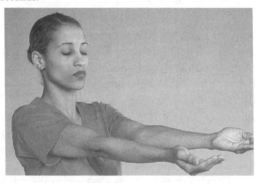

Normal

Your patient should be able to stand with his eyes closed and with his arms straight out without body swaying or arm drifting.

Abnormal

If your patient loses his balance, this indicates a positive Romberg test. This is caused by ataxia from a loss of position sense. If he cannot maintain his balance with his eyes open and feet together, this represents a cerebellar ataxia. If one forearm pronates, suspect a mild hemiparesis. If it drifts sideways or upward, suspect a loss of position sense.

RAPID ALTERNATING MOVEMENTS

Exam

Ask your patient to tap the distal joint of his thumb with the tip of his index finger as rapidly as possible. Then ask him to place his hand, palm up, on his thigh, quickly turn it over palm down, and return it palm up. Have him repeat this movement as quickly as possible for 15 seconds. Evaluate this movement for both hands.

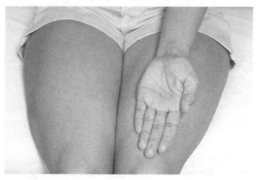

Point-to-point: Ask him to alternate touching your index finger and his nose several times while you observe for accuracy and smoothness.

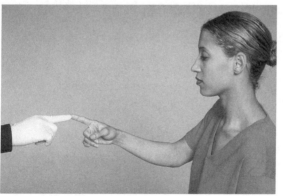

Heel-to-shin: Ask him to place his heel to the opposite knee, then run it down his shin to his big toe.

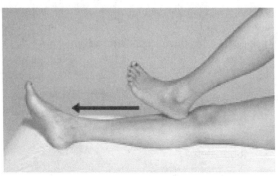

Normal
Your patient should be able to perform these tests with no difficulty.

Abnormal
Keep in mind that his dominant hand usually will perform better than his nondominant hand. If his movements are slow, irregular and clumsy, suspect cerebellar or extra-pyramidal tract disease, or upper motor neuron weakness. Note any tremors or difficulty performing this task, indicating cerebellar disease.

SENSATION

Exam

Test your patient for the following sensations. Remember to compare distal areas to proximal areas, compare symmetrical areas bilaterally, and scatter the stimuli to assess most of the dermatomes.

Pain   Ask your patient to close his eyes. Now touch his skin with a sharp object and ask him to tell you whether it is sharp or dull. Compare areas as you move along the different regions, substituting a dull object for the sharp one intermittently.

Light touch   Ask him to close his eyes; then lightly touch him with a fine piece of cotton. Ask him to respond whenever he feels the cotton.

Temperature   Touch his skin with a vial filled with either hot or cold liquid.

Position   Pull one toe upward and ask your patient to tell you "up" or "down."

Vibration   Place the stem of a vibrating tuning fork against a bony prominence.

Discrimination Put a familiar object, such as a key, into your patient's hand, and ask him to identify it.

Normal

Your patient should exhibit full sensory compliance in all dermatomes.

Abnormal

An abnormality suggests a central or peripheral neuropathy.

Dermatome Chart

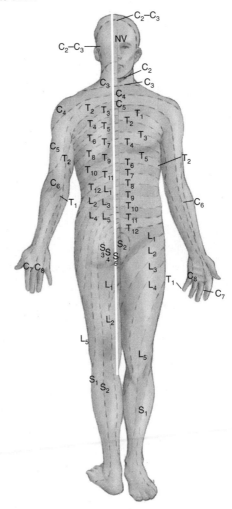

REFLEXES

Exam

To test for deep tendon reflexes, you need a reflex hammer. Use the pointed end for striking small areas and the flat end for striking larger areas. First ask your patient to relax. Then properly position the limb you are testing. Quickly strike the tendon, using wrist motion only. Always compare one side to the other. Grade the reflexes on a scale of 0 to 4+.

BICEPS

Support your patient's arm in the slightly flexed position with your thumb directly over the distal biceps tendon in the antecubital space. Now strike your thumbnail with the point of the reflex hammer and watch for contraction of the biceps muscle and the resulting flexion of the elbow.

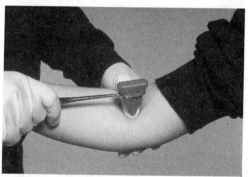

TRICEPS

Flex his arm at a right angle and strike the triceps tendon with the point of your reflex hammer along the posterior aspect of the distal humerus and watch for triceps contraction and the resulting elbow extension.

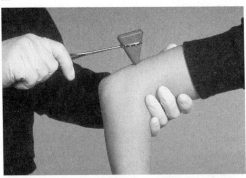

BRACHIORADIALIS

Rest your patient's arm on his leg or lap with the forearm slightly pronated. Now strike his radius about 2 inches above his wrist. Watch for contraction of the brachioradialis muscle and the resulting flexion and supination of the forearm.

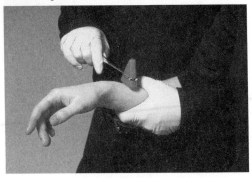

QUADRICEPS

Have your patient sit with his leg hanging off the end of the exam table. Now tap the tendon just below the patella and watch for the quadriceps muscles to contract and extend the knee.

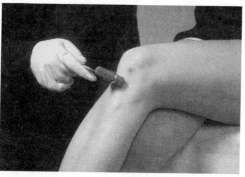

ACHILLES

With your patient sitting, dorsiflex the foot at the ankle and strike the Achilles tendon. Watch for the calf muscles to contract and cause plantar flexion of the foot.

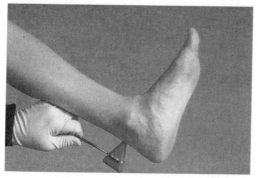

PLANTAR

Stroke the lateral aspect of the sole from the heel to the ball of your patient's foot, curving medially across the ball. Begin with the lightest stimulus that will elicit a response. If no response is detected, be more firm. Watch for plantar flexion of the toes.

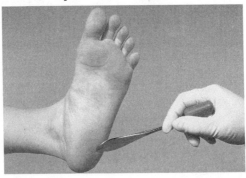

ABDOMINAL

Lightly stroke each side of the abdomen above and below the umbilicus with an irregular object such as a broken Q-tip or a split tongue blade. Note the contraction of the abdominal muscles and how the umbilicus deviates toward the stimulus.

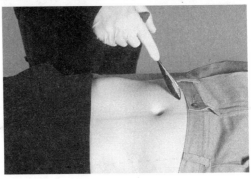

Normal

Your patient should exhibit normal reflexive behavior in all areas.

Reflex Grading Chart

Grade	Description
0	No response
+	Diminished, below normal
+ +	Average, normal
+ + +	Brisker than normal
+ + + +	Hyperreactive, associated with clonus

Abnormal

A diminished or no response suggests damage to the lower motor neurons or spinal cord. A hyperreactive response suggests upper motor neuron disease or injury. When performing the plantar reflex, note if the big toe dorsiflexes while the other toes fan out. This is known as a positive Babinski response, normal in children, and indicates a central nervous system lesion. Absence of abdominal reflexes can suggest either a central or peripheral nervous system disorder.

EMERGENCY FIELD ASSESSMENTS

EMERGENCY FIELD ASSESSMENTS

Conducting a patient assessment in the field involves the following components:

A. Scene Survey
   1. Body substance isolation
   2. Scene safety
   3. Locating all patients
   4. Mechanism of injury
   5. Nature of illness

B. Initial Assessment
   1. General impression
   2. Stabilize cervical spine as needed
   3. Baseline level of response
   4. Airway
   5. Breathing
   6. Circulation
   7. Assign priority

C. Focused History and Physical Exam
   1. Major trauma patient
   2. Minor trauma patient
   3. Responsive medical patient
   4. Unresponsive medical patient

D. Detailed Physical Exam

E. Ongoing Assessment

BODY SUBSTANCE ISOLATION

Disposable gloves should be worn in all cases.

Task	Gown	Mask	Eyewear
Bleeding control with spurting blood	Yes	Yes	Yes
Bleeding control with minimal blood	No	No	No
Childbirth	Yes	Yes	Yes
Drawing blood	No	No	No
Starting an IV	No	No	No
ET Intubation	No	Yes*	Yes
EOA Insertion	No	Yes*	Yes
Suctioning	Yes	Yes*	Yes
Cleaning contaminated instruments	Yes	Yes*	Yes
Taking BP	No	No	No
Giving an injection	No	No	No
Cleaning contaminated ambulance	Yes	Yes	Yes

*HEPA masks should be worn when caring for patients with suspected or confirmed tuberculosis.

EMERGENCY FIELD ASSESSMENTS

TRAUMA TRIAGE CRITERIA

The following mechanisms of injury are predictors of serious internal injury. Quickly transport patients to a trauma center if the mechanism of injury or your patient's clinical condition indicates serious internal injury.

- Ejection from a vehicle
- Fall from greater than 20 feet
- Vehicle rollover
- High-speed collision with severe vehicle deformity
- Vehicle–passenger collision
- Motorcycle crash
- Penetration of the head, chest, or abdomen
- Death of another occupant in the same vehicle

Additional criteria for infants and children include

- Fall from greater than 10 feet
- Bicycle collision
- Medium-speed collision with severe vehicle deformity

EMERGENCY FIELD ASSESSMENTS

INITIAL ASSESSMENT

- Forming a general impression
- Stabilizing the cervical spine as needed
- Assessing baseline mental status
  — AVPU Scale
- Assessing and managing the airway
  — Manual maneuvers
  — Oropharyngeal suctioning
  — Oral/nasal airways
  — Advanced airway procedures as needed
- Assessing and managing breathing
  — Rate, quality, and regularity
  — Positive pressure ventilation
  — Oxygen administration
- Assessing and managing circulation
  — Pulse rate, quality, location, and regularity
  — Hemorrhage control
  — Skin condition
- Determining priority
  — Transport patient immediately
  — Further assess and stabilize patient on scene

EMERGENCY FIELD ASSESSMENTS

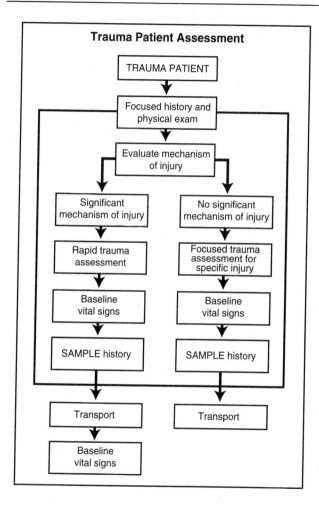

Trauma Patient Assessment

TRAUMA PATIENT
↓
Focused history and physical exam
↓
Evaluate mechanism of injury

Significant mechanism of injury
↓
Rapid trauma assessment
↓
Baseline vital signs
↓
SAMPLE history
↓
Transport
↓
Baseline vital signs

No significant mechanism of injury
↓
Focused trauma assessment for specific injury
↓
Baseline vital signs
↓
SAMPLE history
↓
Transport

EMERGENCY FIELD ASSESSMENTS

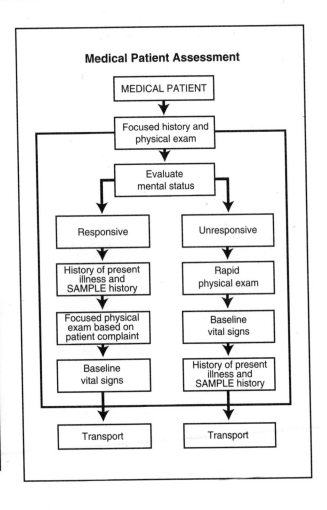

Medical Patient Assessment

MEDICAL PATIENT

↓

Focused history and
physical exam

↓

Evaluate
mental status

Responsive | **Unresponsive**

History of present
illness and
SAMPLE history | Rapid
physical exam

Focused physical
exam based on
patient complaint | Baseline
vital signs

Baseline
vital signs | History of present
illness and
SAMPLE history

Transport | Transport

EMERGENCY FIELD ASSESSMENTS

APPENDICES

PATIENT REPORT FORMAT

- Identify provider, agency, and unit
- Description of scene/mechanism of injury
- Patient's age, sex (if pertinent, race and approximate weight)
- Chief complaint and severity
- Brief, pertinent history of present illness
  - OPQRST-ASPN
- Pertinent past history/current health status/ROS
  - SAMPLE
  - GRAMPS*
- Focused physical exam
  - Head-to-toe survey
  - Tests (ECG, blood sugar, pulse ox)
- Treatments administered/request for orders
- Estimated time of arrival (ETA)

*GRAMPS is a helpful mnemonic for eliciting a history from responsive patients during a medical emergency:

G	Genetics (family history)
R	Recreational drugs (smoking, alcohol, drugs)
A	Allergies
M	Medications
P	Past medical history
S	Social history

APPENDICES

CHARTING ABBREVIATIONS

Patient Information/Categories

Asian	A
Black	B
Chief complaint	C
Complains of	c/o
Current health status	CHS
Date of birth	DOB
Differential diagnosis	DD
Estimated time of confinement	EDC
Family History	FH
Female	♀
Hispanic	H
History	Hx
History and physical	H&P
History of present illness	HPI
Impression	IMP
Male	♂
Medications	Med
Newborn	NB
Occupational history	OH
Past history	PH
Patient	Pt
Physical exam	PE
Private medical doctor	PMD
Review of systems	ROS
Signs and symptoms	S&S
Social history	SH

Visual acuity	VA
Vital signs	VS
Weight	Wt
White	W
Year-old	y/o

Body Systems

Abdomen	Abd
Cardiovascular	CV
Central nervous	CNS
Ear, nose, and throat	ENT
Gastrointestinal	GI
Genitourinary	GU
Gynecological	GYN
Head, eyes, ears, nose, throat	HEENT
Musculoskeletal	M/S
Obstetrical	OB
Peripheral nervous	PNS
Respiratory	Resp

Common Complaints

Abdominal pain	abd pn
Chest pain	CP
Dyspnea on exertion	DOE
Fever of unknown origin	FUO
Gunshot wound	GSW
Headache	H/A
Lower back pain	LBP
Nausea/vomiting	n/v

No apparent distress	NAD
Pain	pn
Shortness of breath	SOB
Substernal chest pain	SSCP

Diagnoses

Abdominal aortic aneurysm	AAA
Abortion	Ab
Acute myocrdial infarction	AMI
Adult respiratory distress syndrome	ARDS
Alcohol	ETOH
Atherosclerotic heart disease	ASHD
Chronic obstructve pulmonary disease	COPD
Chronic renal failure	CRF
Congestive heart failure	CHF
Coronary artery bypass graft	CABG
Coronary artery disease	CAD
Cystic fibrosis	CF
Dead on arrival	DOA
Delirium tremens	DTs
Deep vein thrombosis	DVT
Diabetes mellitus	DM
Dilation and curettage	D&C
Duodenal ulcer	DU
End-stage renal failure	ESRF
Epstein-Barr virus	EBF
Foreign body obstruction	FBO
Hepatitis B virus	HBV
Hiatal hernia	HH

Hypertension	HTN
Infectious disease	ID
Inferior wall myocardial infarction	IWMI
Insulin-dependent diabetes mellitus	IDDM
Intracranial pressure	ICP
Mass casualty incident	MCI
Mitral valve prolapse	MVP
Motor vehicle crash	MVC
Multiple sclerosis	MS
Non-insulin-dependent diabetes mellitus	NIDDM
Organic brain syndrome	OBS
Otitis media	OM
Overdose	OD
Paroxysmal nocturnal dyspnea	PND
Pelvic inflammatory disease	PID
Peptic ulcer disease	PUD
Pregnancies/births (gravida/para)	G/P
Pregnancy-induced hypertension	PIH
Pulmonary embolism	PE
Rheumatic heart disease	RHD
Sexually transmitted disease	STD
Transient ischemic attack	TIA
Tuberculosis	TB
Upper respiratory infection	URI
Urinary tract infection	UTI
Venereal disease	VD
Wolff-Parkinson-White syndrome	WPW

Angiotensin-converting enzyme	ACE
Aspirin	ASA
Bicarbonate	HCO3
Birth control pills	BCP
Calcium	Ca++
Calcium channel blocker	CCB
Calcium chloride	CaCl2
Chloride	Cl–
Digoxin	Dig
Dilantin (phenytoin sodium)	DPH
Diphenhydramine	DPHM
Diptheria-Pertussis-Tetanus	DPT
Hydrochlorothiazide	HCTZ
Lactated Ringer's/Ringer's Lactate	LR/RL
Magnesium sulfate	Mg++
Morphine sulfate	MS
Nitroglycerine	NTG
Nonsteroidal antiinflammatory drug	NSAID
Normal saline	NS
Penicillin	PCN
Phenobarbital	PB
Potassium	K+
Sodium bicarbonate	NaHCO3
Sodium chloride	NaCl
Tylenol	APAP

APPENDICES

Abdomen	Abd
Antecubital	AC
Anterior axillary line	AAL
Anterior cruciate ligament	ACL
Anterior–posterior	A/P
Distal interphalangeal (joint)	DIP
Dorsalis pedis (pulse)	DP
Gallbladder	GB
Intercostal space	ICS
Lateral collateral ligament	LCL
Left lower lobe	LLL
Left lower quadrant	LLQ
Left upper lobe	LUL
Left upper quadrant	LUQ
Left ventricle	LV
Liver, spleen, kidneys	LSK
Lymph node	LN
Medial collateral ligament	MCL
Metacarpalphalangeal (joint)	MCP
Metatarsalphalangeal (joint)	MTP
Midaxillary line	MAL
Posterior axillary line	PAL
Posterior cruciate ligament	PCL
Right lower lobe	RLL
Right lower quadrant	RLQ
Right middle lobe	RML
Right upper lobe	RUL

Right upper quadrant	RUQ
Temporomandibular joint	TMJ
Tympanic membrane	TM

Physical Exam/Findings

Arterial bloood gas	ABG
Bilateral breath sounds	BBS
Blood sugar	BS
Breath sounds	BS
Cardiac injury profile	CIP
Central venous pressure	CVP
Cerebrospinal fluid	CSF
Chest X-ray	CXR
Complete blood count	CBC
Computerized tomography	CT
Conscious, alert, oriented	CAO
Costovertebral angle	CVA
Deep tendon reflexes	DTR
Dorsalis pedis	DP
Electrocardiogram	ECG, EKG
Electroencephalogram	EEG
Expiratory	Exp
Extraoccular movements (intact)	EOM(I)
Fetal heart tones	FHT
Full range of motion	FROM
Full-term normal delivery	FTND
Heart rate	HR
Heart sounds	HS
Heel-to-shin	H → S

Hemoglobin	Hgb
Inspiratory	Insp
Jugular venous distention	JVD
Laceration	lac
Level of consciousness	LOC
Moves all extremities (well)	MAE (W)
Nontender	NT
Normal range of motion	NROM
Palpation	Palp
Passive range of motion	PROM
Point of maximal impulse	PMI
Posterior tibial	PT
Pulse	P
Pupils equal, round, reactive to light and accommodation	PERRLA
Range of motion	ROM
Respirations	R
Tactile vocal fremitus	TVF
Temperature	T
Unconscious	unc
Urinary incontinence	UI

Miscellaneous

After (post)	$\bar{p}$
After eating	pc
Alert and oriented	A/O
Anterior	ant.
Approximate	$\approx$
As needed	prn

Before (ante)	$\bar{a}$
Before eating (ante cibum)	$\bar{a}.c.$
Body surface area	BSA
Celcius	C°
Change	Δ
Decreased	↓
Equal	=
Fahrenheit	F°
Immediately	stat
Increased	↑
Inferior	inf.
Left	L
Less than	<
Moderate	mod.
More than	>
Negative	–
No, not, none	∅
Not applicable	n/a
Number	no, #
Occasional	occ
Pack years	pk/yrs
Per	/
Positive	+
Posterior	post.
Postoperative	PO
Prior to arrival	PTA
Radiates to	⟶
Right	R

Rule out	R/O
Secondary to	2°
Superior	sup.
Times (for 3 hrs)	x (x3h)
Unequal	≠
Warm and dry	W/D
While awake	WA
With (cum)	$\bar{c}$
Within normal limits	WNL
With (cum)	$\bar{s}$
Zero	∅

Treatments/Dispositions

Advanced cardiac life support	ACLS
Advanced life support	ALS
Against medical advice	AMA
Automated external defibrillator	AED
Bag-valve-mask	BVM
Basic life support	BLS
Cardiopulmonary resuscitation	CPR
Carotid sinus massage	CSM
Continuous positive airway pressure	CPAP
Do not resuscitate	DNR
Endotracheal tube	ETT
Estimated time of arrival	ETA
External cardiac pacing	ECP
Intermittent positive pressure ventilation	IPPV
Long spine board	LSB
Nasal cannula	NC

Nasogastric	NG
Nasopharyngeal airway	NPA
No transport–refusal	NTR
Nonrebreather mask	NRM, NRB
Nothing by mouth	NPO
Occupational therapy	OT
Oropharyngeal airway	OPA
Oxygen	O_2
Per square inch	psi
Physical therapy	PT
Positive-end expiratory pressure	PEEP
Short spine board	SSB
Therapy	Rx
Treatment	Tx
Turned over to	TOT
Verbal order	VO

Medication Administration/Metrics

Centimeter	cm
Cubic centimeter	cc
Deciliter	dL
Drop(s)	gtt(s)
Drops per minute	gtts/min
Every	q
Grain	gr
Gram	g, gm
Hour	h, hr
Hydrogen-ion concentration	pH
Intracardiac	IC

Intramuscular	IM
Intraosseous	IO
Intravenous	IV
Intravenous push	IVP
Joules	j
Keep vein open	KVO
Kilogram	kg
Liter	L
Liters per minute	L/min
Microgram	mcg
Milliequivalent	mEq
Milligram	mg
Milliliter	ml
Millimeter	mm
Millimeters of mercury	mmHg
Minute	min
Orally	po
Subcutaneous	SC, SQ
To keep open	TKO

Cardiology

Atrial fibrillation	AF
Atrial tachycardia	AT
Atrioventricular	AV
Bundle branch block	BBB
Complete heart block	CHB
Electromechanical dissociation	EMD
Idioventricular rhythm	IVR
Junctional rhythm	JR

Modified chest lead	MCL
Multifacial atrial tachycardia	MAT
Normal sinus rhythm	NSR
Paroxysmal supraventricular tachycardia	PSVT
Premature atrial contraction	PAC
Premature junctional contraction	PJC
Premature ventricular contraction	PVC
Pulseless electrical activity	PEA
Supraventricular tachycardia	SVT
Ventricular tachycardia	VT
Ventricular fibrillation	VF
Wandering atrial pacemaker	WAP

APPENDICES

PATIENT REFUSAL CHECKLIST

Before allowing your patient to refuse care and transport against your advice, go through this checklist and document the information on your PCR.

- Have you done a thorough assessment of your patient?
- Is your patient competent to refuse care?
- Did you recommend care and transport?
- Did you explain to your patient about possible consequences of refusing care, including possibility of death, if appropriate?
- Have you offered other suggestions for accessing care?
- Have you expressed a willingness to return if your patient changes his mind?
- Does your patient understand your statements and suggestions, and is he apparently competent to refuse care based on that understanding?
- Has your patient signed the refusal block on the DCR?

SOAP FORMAT

Subjective

- Chief complaint
- History of present illness
- Past history
- Current health status
- Review of systems

Objective

- Vital signs
- General impression
- Physical exam
- Diagnostic tests

Assessment

- Field diagnosis

Plan

- Standing orders
- Physician orders
- Effects of interventions
- Mode of transportation
- Ongoing assessment

CHIEF COMPLAINT
History

- History of present illness
- Past history
- Current health status
- Review of systems

Assessment

- Vital signs
- General impression
- Physical exam
- Diagnostic tests
- Field diagnosis

Rx

- Standing orders
- Physician orders

Transport

- Effects of interventions
- Mode of transportation
- Ongoing assessment

APGAR SCORE

Criterion	0	1	2
Heart rate	Absent	< 100	> 100
Respiration	Absent	Slow/irregular	Good cry
Muscle tone	Limp	Some flexion	Active motion
Reflex/irritability	None	Grimace	Vigorous cough
Color	Blue/pale	Ext blue/body pink	Pink

GLASGOW COMA SCORE

Eye Opening

	Infant	Adult	
4	Spontaneously	Spontaneously	4
3	To command	To speech	3
2	To pain	To pain	2
1	None	None	1

Best Verbal Response

5	Coos, babbles, smiles	Oriented	5
4	Irritable, cries	Confused	4
3	Cries, screams to pain	Inappropriate words	3
2	Moans, grunts	Incomprehensible sounds	2
1	None	None	1

Best Motor Response

6	Spontaneous	Obeys command	6
5	Withdraws from touch	Localizes pain	5
4	Withdraws from pain	Withdraws from pain	4
3	Flexion (decorticate)	Flexion (decorticate)	3
2	Extension (decerebrate)	Extension (decerebrate)	2
1	None	None	1

BURNS

Burn Chart

Body Area	Infant	Child	Adult
Head	18	18	9
Chest and abdomen	18	18	18
Back	18	18	18
Arms	9	9	9
Legs	14	14	18

Critical Burns

Adult

- Respiratory burns
- Partial or full thickness burns to the face, feet, hands
- Full thickness burns of > 10%
- Partial thickness burns of >30%
- Burns complicated by musculoskeletal injuries
- Circumferential burns
- Burns in the presence of significant underlying medical illness

Pediatric

- Full or partial thickness burns of > 20%

S.T.A.R.T. TRIAGE ALGORITHM

Step 1—Move all walking wounded to a safe area for care.

Step 2—Leave all dead or mortally wounded for medical examiner.

Step 3—Begin S.T.A.R.T. triage method for all other victims:

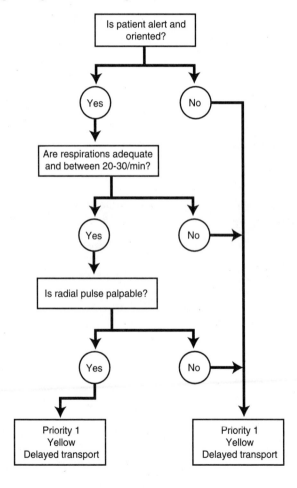

APPENDICES

INDEX

See also Charting Abbreviations on pages 133-145.